Awareness and Knowledge about Disposal of Unused and Expired Medication among Professionals and Students

Research Team

- Dr. Snehalata D. Ghatol (Principal Investigator)

Survey Team- Trainee Teachers

- Ms. Payal Rathod,
- Ms. Megha Patel,
- Ms. Deepika Chauhan,
- Ms. Divya Parekh

Prepared by

- Dr. Snehalata D. Ghatol (Principal Investigator)

Funding

- No funding was obtained for the conduct of this research

Conflict of interest

- None

Ethical approval

- The study was approved by the Institutional Authorities

Disclaimers

- With an aim to present observations and practises followed in disposal of unused and date expired medicines across globe, information on rules and regulations were compiled from published sources. In order not to change its medical meaning, they are produced as it in the report and are cited and acknowledge properly at appropriate places.
- The view expressed by the authors is her own and not related to the organisation she attached with.

Published by

Draft Project Completed in March 2025
Final Report Published in March 2025

Citation

Ghatol Snehalata D. (2025). Study of Awareness and Knowledge about Disposal of Unused and Expired Medication among Professionals and Students, Sardar Patel College of Education, Sardar Patel Education Campus, Bakrol 388315, Anand, Gujarat (India).

Awareness and Knowledge about Disposal of Unused and Expired Medication among Professionals and Students

Dr. Snehalata Ghatol

ALLIED PUBLISHERS PVT. LTD.

Noida • Mumbai • Kolkata • Chennai • Bangalore

ALLIED PUBLISHERS PRIVATE LIMITED

D-5, Sector-2, **Noida**–201 301
Ph. Nos.: 0120-4320295/2542557/4352866 • E-mail: delhi.books@alliedpublishers.com

17 Chittaranjan Avenue, **Kolkata**–700072
Ph.: 033-22129618 • E-mail: cal.books@alliedpublishers.com

15 J.N. Heredia Marg, Ballard Estate, **Mumbai**–400001
Ph.: 022-42126969 • E-mail: mumbai.books@alliedpublishers.com

No. 25/10, Commander-in-Chief Road, Ethiraj Lane (Next to Post Office)
Egmore, **Chennai**–600008
Ph.: 044-28223938 • E-mail: chennai.books@alliedpublishers.com

P.B. No. 9932, No. 15, 3rd Floor (Next to Vijaya Bank), 5th Cross, Gandhinagar,
Karnataka, **Bangalore**–560009, Ph.: 080-41530285 / 22386239
E-mail: bngl.books@alliedpublishers.com

Website: www.alliedpublishers.com

ISBN: 978-93-89934-81-6

Published by Sunil Sachdev and printed by Ravi Sachdev at Allied Publishers Pvt. Ltd.,
D-5, Sector-2, Noida–201 301

Foreword

Medicine is important because it can treat and prevent diseases, relieve pain, and improve quality of life. Access to medicine is a cornerstone of public health and an effective indicator of social equality. However, medicines can also have risks if not used safely. Safe use of medicine includes safe storage and disposal. It is crucial that we organize and keep track of the drugs that we use. Drug disposal is the discarding of drugs. People generally dispose of unused drugs that remain after the end of medical treatment. Health care organizations dispose of drugs on a larger scale for a various reason, including having leftover drugs after treating patients and discarding of expired drugs. Failure to proper disposal of drugs creates opportunities for others (of whom the drug is unintended) to take them inappropriately. Inappropriate disposal of drugs can also cause drug pollution. People dispose of drugs in numerous ways. Even though organizations have expertise on drugs, they give inconsistent information about drug disposal to the consumers. Expired drugs should be disposed off safely, without causing harm to the people and the environment. Improper medicine disposal poses environmental and public health risks, with common methods like flushing or throwing in the trash being detrimental. Pollution has been a challenge for sustainable development and pharmaceutical pollution has direct implications in the environmental, economic and social spheres, which are considered the triad for sustainable development. There has been no study regarding the disposal practices of unwanted pharmaceutical products conducted in Gujarat. The results of these studies are necessary for developing effective measures to increase public awareness of medication disposal and the harms associated with its improper practices.

This report provides the field survey research on awareness and knowledge concerning the correct disposal of unused and expired drugs among professional, student and households in Gujarat on reach and benefit of program in the state of Gujarat. The study is primarily based on primary data. The study was conducted in the state of Gujarat covering the 385 respondents from rural, semi-urban and urban areas of Gujarat.

The study observed that consumers had poor knowledge regarding the safe drug disposal techniques. Therefore, it is the need of the hour to take stringent actions and formulate uniform guidelines on the safe disposal of medicines. Moreover, safe disposal instructions should be provided by all healthcare providers to patients in routine practice. Thus, efforts need to be done by every section of the society for the safe disposal of medications in order to create a safe environment for future.

I would like to congratulate Dr Snehalata Ghatol madam and entire project team for preparing this excellent research report. I hope findings of the study would be useful for academicians, policy makers and researchers.

Dr. Prabhat Kasra
Principal
Sardar Patel College of Education,
Sardar Patel Education Campus,
Bakrol 388315, Anand, Gujarat (India)

Acknowledgements

The study on "**Awareness and Knowledge about Disposal of Unused and Expired Medication among Professionals and Students**" has been carried out at Sardar Patel College of Education, Sardar Patel Education Campus, Bakrol 388315, Anand, Gujarat (India) as a minor research project.

I have benefited immensely from various scholars and officials from different institutions and departments while carrying out this study. At the outset, we would like to thank **Shri Girish Patel**, Chairman, Tirupati Foundation Trust, Bakrol; **Shri Shital D. Patel**, Secretary, Tirupati Foundation Trust, Bakrol for their encouragement and guidance in undertaking this research study. I also thank **Dr. Forum Patel** (Campus Coordinator) and **Shri Dhiren Patel** (Administrative Head) for their support.

I am thankful to **Dr. Prabhat Kasara**, Principal, SPCE (B.Ed), **Dr. Arti Patel** (IQAC Coordinator) and all my colleagues in college for their necessary support during survey work of this project.

I am grateful to **Dr. Kinjal Ahir**, Head, post Graduate Department of Economics, Sardar Patel University, Vallabh Vidyanagar for sharing this topic of research and providing necessary insights on the topic.

I also thank **Dr. Neepa Bharucha**, Associate Professor, M.B. Patel College of Education, Sardar Patel University, Vallabh Vidyanagar for her guidance in framing the schedules and providing constructive comments on draft report.

I also thank our Trainee Teachers (**Ms. Payal Rathod, Ms. Megha Patel, Ms. Deepika Chauhan, Mr. Divya Parekh**) for their support during survey work of this project. I also thank all of them who have directly and indirectly helped in conducting this study.

The study would not have reached to this stage without the active co-operation of the sample respondents (Students, Pharmacists and others), who provided all the required data for the study without any hesitation and expectation. We thank each one of them for their invaluable support.

I have also received support and encouragements from our colleagues in the SPCE (B.Ed) while carrying out the study.

Lastly but not least, we thank all the staff of SPCE (B.Ed) staff for their direct and indirect support.

Sardar Patel College of Education,
Sardar Patel Education Campus,
Bakrol 388315, Anand, Gujarat
(India)

Dr. Snehalata D. Ghatol
Assistant Professor

Content

List of Tables

List of Figures

List of Maps

List of Annexures

List of Abbreviations

APL	:	Above Poverty Line
Av.	:	Average
B. Pharm	:	Bachelor of Pharmacy
B.Ed.	:	Bachelor of Education
BPL	:	Below Poverty Line
CPCB	:	Central Pollution Control Board
D. Pharm	:	Diploma of Pharmacy
DGCI	:	Drug Controller General of India
GMP	:	Good Manufacturing Practices
GoI	:	Government of India
NCB	:	Narcotics Control Bureau
NFI	:	National Formulary of India
NHM	:	National Health Mission
OBC	:	Other Backward Classes
OECD	:	Organization for Economic Co-operation and Development
SC	:	Scheduled Caste
ST	:	Scheduled Tribe
US	:	United State
WHO	:	World Health Organisation

Awareness and Knowledge about Disposal of Unused and Expired Medication among Professionals and Students

Dr. Snehalata D. Ghatol

Medicines play a very significant role for treating many diseases and conditions, but at the end of the treatment it is very important to dispose them of properly. So, the knowledge and awareness of proper drug disposal are essential for safe environment. In the modern era, with the improved methods of development of new medications, more and more efficacious and safe medicines have been marketed to treat diverse diseased states. At the same time, the risk of contamination of the environment with the increased usage of medicines in humans and in veterinarians has been increased manifold. The common preventive step to protect the environment from this kind of pharmaceutical waste is by creating the awareness about proper disposal method to avoid the pollution of environment and their impacts. the main objective of the study is to find out the knowledge, general practices, awareness, concerning the correct disposal of unused and expired drugs among healthcare professionals and student households in Gujarat. The data were collected through personal interview method from 400 (385 respondents + 15 pharmacists). The study observed that consumers had poor knowledge regarding the safe drug disposal techniques. Therefore, it is the need of the hour to take stringent actions and formulate uniform guidelines on the safe disposal of medicines. Moreover, safe disposal instructions should be provided by all healthcare providers to patients in routine practice. Thus, efforts need to be done by every section of the society for the safe disposal of medications in order to create a safe environment for future.

Keywords: *Medication Disposal, Unused Medicines, Expired Medicines.*

Acknowledgements

The author would like to acknowledge respondents and students for their invaluable contributions.

CHAPTER I

Introduction

1.1 Introduction

Medicines play a very significant role for treating many diseases and conditions. Humankind life expectancy has been increasing with the advance of medicine and therefore pharmaceutical industry is essential for human health. The growth of the pharmaceutical industry and better access to medications all contribute to a rise in drug use and accumulation in households throughout the World (Toe, *et al.*, 2023). Medicine consumption is increasing day by day all over the world, especially in countries like India and China (Figure 1.1). Global use of medicines grew by 14 per cent over the past five years (2020–2024) and a further 12 per cent increase is expected through 2028, bringing annual use to 3.8 trillion defined daily doses (GUM, 2024). The highest volume growth over the next five years is expected in China, India and Asia-Pacific, all exceeding 3 per cent compound annual growth. The corona-virus pandemic has increased prescription drug use and impacted the way people get their medications.

India is the populous country in the world having 1.45 billion populations (2024). India's pharmaceutical industry is the third largest by volume after China and Italy. Medicine consumption is associated with population growth and their environmental occurrence has implications for human and environmental health (Quadra *et al.*, 2017; Klatte *et al.*, 2017). The medicines consumption generally increases while humans are getting old since the immunological system does not work at the same efficiency and the incidence of chronic diseases enhances. In India, both the share and size of elderly population is increasing over time. From 5.6 per cent in 1961, the proportion has increased to 8.6 per cent in 2011. The proportion has increased to 10.1 per cent in 2021 and further likely to increase to 13.1 per cent in 2031. India is ageing rapidly, sixty plus will make up 15 per cent of population by 2036. Besides, share of expenditure on medicines as part of the total out-of-pocket (OOP) expenditure on healthcare services has been reported to be much higher in India than in other countries (Prinja *et al.*, 2022). With India on the brink of a demographic shift, the care and well-being of its senior citizens must become a national priority.

Historical and projected use of medicines by region, 2018–2028, Defined Daily Doses (DDD) in billions.

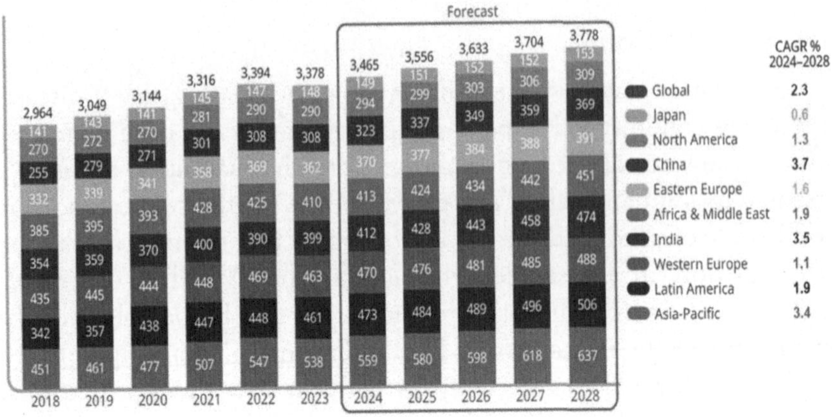

Figure 1.1: Historical and Projected Use of Medicines by Region (2018–2028)

Notes: Chart represents IQVIA Institute estimates of global defined daily doses (DDD). These estimates are based on IQVIA audited data and application of WHO-DDD factors in IQVIA MIDAS as well as additional DDD calculation assumptions developed by the IQVIA Institute (see Methodology). Asia-Pacific does not include China, India, and Japan which are reported separately. 2023 volume is based on actual data as of June 2023 and projected for the remainder of the year.

Report: Global Use of Medicines 2024: Outlook to 2028. IQVIA Institute for Human Data Science, January 2024.

Source: IQVIA Institute, Dec 2023.
https://www.iqvia.com

Since disease incidence and prevalence have been rising over the past few decades, especially from COVID-19, healthcare practitioners must prescribe and dispense numerous medications. Though, more emphasis is made on the rational use of medicine such that patients should receive the right medicines at the right time and use them appropriately. While irrational use of medicines (overuse, underuse or misuse of medicines) results in wastage of scarce resources and widespread health hazards is a major problem worldwide. Most of the time, these prescribed medicines are left unused due to various reasons like the change of treatment, side effects of the drug, improvement of patient condition resulting in discontinuation of the course of treatment, adverse effects, dosage adjustment, recovery from disease, expiration date, physician prescribing practice, dispenser practice, and so forth (Abahussain, 2012). In addition, storage of unused medicine at home may increase the risk of a wide range of potential drug-related problems like errors in taking medications, adverse drug reactions, and can be considered as a waste of resources. Unused, unwanted, and expired drugs kept at home endanger both health systems and the environment (Sarraf *et al.,* 2022 A survey conducted on over 33,000 respondents by Local Circles says people throw away anything between 10 per cent and 70 per cent of the medicines bought/ prescribe. About 50 per cent of people surveyed say pharmacists sell a higher minimum quantity than what is required. About 29 per cent of respondents say that they stopped taking the prescribed dosage once they were on the mend[1]. Eventually these medicines are disposed-off but there is a lacuna in proper disposal practices. Improper disposal of medicines can cause an environmental contamination which leads to health hazards.

1.2 Environmental Pollution through Improper Disposal of Medicines

In the last decade, the disposal of unused or expired pharmaceuticals has gained a particular interest. The global increase in pharmaceutical spending has led to an enhanced international awareness on the issue of unused medications and harmful economic, environmental and health effects of improper medicine disposal (Braund *et al.,* 2009; EEA 2010; Kummerer 2008). It is important to dispose the medicines that are date expired and unused in an appropriate manner. The incorrect disposal of medicines in trash, toilets or sinks, as well as industrial effluents and veterinary application, are other potential sources of pharmaceuticals to the environment (Quadra *et al.*, 2017; Klatte *et al.*, 2017). Currently, a high amount of pharmaceutical wastes flows through sewerage into the water bodies alarming the environmental scientist around the world and are also getting absorbed into the land when they are disposed of as solid waste in landfills. It was established that tons of municipal solid waste are generated due to expired and unused drugs. These are due to the improper disposal of unused medications through environmentally-unfriendly routes. To overcome this problem the proper handling of the expired drugs is

[1] https://www.business-standard.com

imperative. Moreover, the improper drug disposal causes various consequences like accidental consumption of expired drugs, resale or misuse during sorting. Thus, non-rational use of medicines as well as non-awareness about disposal of unused and expired medicines may harm environmental health with the potential to cause public health issues. Thus, after use of prescribed medicine and at the end of the treatment, it is very important to dispose them of properly.

Improper disposal of expired and unused medications has several consequences such as environmental pollution, childhood poisoning, negative impact on wildlife, and development of drug-resistant microorganisms (Michael, *et al.*, 2019). Throwing household expired medicines into the garbage cans or the sewage system can cause environmental hazards that may have implications on public health since some of the medicines consist of potentially harmful ingredients that may accumulate in the environment (Barnett-Itzhaki *et al.*, 2016). When unused medicines are dumped in the environment with municipal rubbish, the active chemicals in the medicines pose harm to the environment and human health because they may be released into the air when the waste is burned or seep into the ground in the presence of water (Toe, *et al.*, 2023). Some classes of returned medicines go through incineration, which depends on each country's regulation. However, open burning is still a common practice, mainly in developing countries, where the waste is not separate at all. Open burning of healthcare waste is a potential source of carbon and other contaminants such as dioxins and furans (WHO 1999; Babanyara *et al.*, 2013; Raila 2017). Black carbon, for example, may intensify global warming due to its capacity to absorb solar energy and increase dark cloud formation, decreasing its ability to reflect sunlight (DeAngelis 2011). So, the knowledge and awareness of proper drug disposal are essential for safe environment. The common preventive step to protect the environment from this kind of pharmaceutical waste is by creating the awareness about proper disposal method to avoid the pollution of environment and their impacts.

1.3 Medicine Disposal Methods

It has been discovered that the general public lacks sufficient understanding of how to dispose of unutilized, unneeded, and expired pharmaceuticals (Medhi & Sewal, 2012). The studies have reported that most Indian households possessed unwanted medicines. This included antibiotics, hormonal medicines, analgesics, anti-hypertensives, antidiabetics, etc. Non-adherence, discontinuation due to side effects, early recovery, etc, are the reasons for unwanted medicines in the households. While analysing the disposal practices, it was found that more than half of the respondents used to dispose-off these unwanted medicines with household garbage (Kaladharan *et al.,* 2023). Previously, it was thought that disposing of any expired or unused prescribed medications in the toilet or down the drain was the best way to prevent accidental intake rather than dumping them in the garbage, where humans or animals were more likely to come into contact with them. As the public became more aware of the potential environmental and public health consequences of medicine flushing, guidelines for pharmaceutical disposal procedures began to evolve (Dar *et al.*, 2019). At different levels, from households to health facilities, the disposal of unfit pharmaceuticals, for instance flushing them down the drain, poses an environmental risk (Persson *et al.*, 2009). Unfortunately, most people flush unneeded pharmaceuticals down the toilet or throw them away in the trash. Some people distribute their prescription drugs to family members or friends (Naser *et al.*, 2021). Many pharmaceutical contaminants have been found in groundwaters, surface waters, seawater, soils, and sludges. When home medications are disposed of in the garbage, solid pharmaceuticals end up in landfills, and liquid pharmaceuticals end up in the environment via liquid drainage systems (Bound & Voulvoulis, 2005).

According to a review of multiple research studies, the most typical manner of disposing of drugs in South Asian nations is through the trash or dustbin. Secondly, the practice of flushing medications down sinks or toilets is also common in countries like India, Pakistan, Indonesia, Malaysia, and Bangladesh. Most critically, the tendency to return unused and expired medicine to pharmacies for appropriate disposal is rarely seen (Table 1.1). The different types of pharmaceuticals disposal method suggested by WHO are presented in Table 1.2.

Table 1.1: Methods of Handling Leftover/Expired Medication in Different Countries

Region	*Method of disposal*				
	Dustin or Trash	*Sink or Toilet*	*Other(s)*	*Returning to Pharmacy*	*References*
Nepal	72%	21%	–	2%	Sarraf, *et al.*, (2022)
Malaysia	84%	12%	–	5%	Azmi & Shakeel (2020)
India	73%	20%	–	–	Manocha, *et al.* (2020)
Pakistan	83%	12%	–	2%	Ahmed & Mushtaq (2013)
Indonesia	82%	5%	4% burned the medicine	0.2%	Insani *et al.*, (2020)
Bangladesh	47%	–	2% burned the medicine	21%	Begum, *et al.*, (2021)

Source: Borhan Uddin, M., Al Samir, R., & Golam Mehebub Pantho, G.M. (2024).

Table 1.2: Different Types of Pharmaceutical Disposal Methods

Disposal Methods	*Types of Pharmaceutical*	*Comments*
Return to donor or manufacturer, transfrontier transfer for disposal	All bulk waste pharmaceuticals, particularly antineoplastics.	Usually not practical - transfrontier procedures may be time consuming.
High temperature incineration with temperatures greatly in excess of 1200°C.	Solids, semisolids, powders, antineoplastics, controlled substances.	Expensive, particularly for purpose-built incinerators. Use of existing industrial plants may be more practical.
Medium temperature incineration with two–chamber incinerator with minimum temperature of 850°C. Cement kiln incineration	In the absence of high temperature incinerators, solids, semi-solids, powders. Controlled substances.	Antineoplastics best incinerated at high temperature.

Disposal Methods	*Types of Pharmaceutical*	*Comments*
Immobilization Waste encapsulation	Solids, semi-solids, powders, liquids, antineoplastics, controlled substances.	
Inertization	Solids, semi-solids, powders, antineoplastics, controlled substances.	
Landfill Highly engineered sanitary landfill	Limited quantities of untreated solids, semi-solids and powders. Disposal of waste pharmaceuticals after immobilization preferable. PVC plastics.	
Engineered landfill	Waste solids, semi-solids and powders, preferably after immobilization. PVC plastics.	
Open uncontrolled non-engineered dump	As last resort untreated solids, semi- solids, powders – must be covered immediately with municipal waste. Immobilization of solids, semi solids, powders is preferable.	Not for untreated controlled substances.
Sewer	Diluted liquids, syrups, intravenous fluids, small quantities of diluted disinfectants (supervised).	Antineoplastics, and undiluted disinfectants & antiseptics not recommended.
Fast–flowing watercourse	Diluted liquids, syrups, intravenous fluids; small quantities of diluted disinfectants (supervised).	Antineoplastics, and undiluted disinfectants and antiseptics not recommended.
Burning in open containers	As last resort, packaging, paper, cardboard.	Not acceptable for PVC plastics or pharmaceuticals.
Chemical decomposition	Not recommended unless special chemical expertise and materials available.	Not practical for quantities over 50 kg.

Source: WHO (1999).

According to the Government of India (GOI) guidelines, the preferred method for disposing of expired or unused medicines is to return them to the manufacturer whenever possible, and for most other cases, to dispose of them as biomedical waste through a designated common bio-medical waste treatment facility, which typically involves proper segregation, packaging, and incineration at high temperatures; with specific care needed for hazardous drugs like cytotoxics. Key points about GoI guidelines for medicine disposal:

- **Biomedical Waste Management Rules:** The primary governing document for medicine disposal is the Bio-Medical Waste Management Rules, which mandates proper segregation and treatment of pharmaceutical waste as part of biomedical waste.
- **Return to Manufacturer:** This is considered the most environmentally sound method, as manufacturers can often recycle components of the medicine.
- **Incineration:** For medicines that cannot be returned, incineration at high temperatures is the recommended disposal method, especially for potent or hazardous drugs.
- **Segregation and Packaging:** Medicines should be properly segregated based on their hazard level and packaged in appropriate containers before disposal.
- **No Flushing:** Flushing medicines down the toilet is not recommended due to potential environmental contamination.
- **Public Awareness:** The government also emphasizes educating the public about proper medicine disposal practices to prevent improper disposal at home.
- **Central Pollution Control Board** (CPCB): Guidelines for Common Bio-Medical Waste Treatment Facilities.
- **Drugs and Cosmetics Act, 1940:** The primary legislation governing drug manufacturing and sale in India.
- **National Health Mission** (NHM): Operational guidelines for drug management and disposal.

1.4 Need of the Study

Unused and expired medicines are potentially toxic substances that should be managed effectively to avoid possible environmental hazards. The absence of well-defined protocols in India regarding the proper disposal of unused, unwanted, and expired medications raises concerns about the potential for accidental poisoning and environmental threats. The accumulation of unused and expired medicines in households and their disposal practices are serious global challenges that need to be investigated.

India continues to have the persisting environmental problem of disposal of expired, unused, unwanted medicines. Since this has not been studied well, the exact repercussions, therefore, are not hitherto known fully. There has been no study regarding the disposal practices of unwanted pharmaceutical products conducted in Gujarat. The results of these studies are necessary for developing effective measures to increase public awareness of medication disposal and the harms associated with its improper practices. Although the National Formulary of India (2016[2] and 2021[3]), specifies guidelines for the proper disposal of medicines, yet most of the people are not aware of these guidelines and the importance to follow them. As this is an emerging issue of concern, the present study was planned to carry out.

1.5 Research Questions

Some of the questions pertaining to the disposal of unused pharmaceuticals by households and individuals include:

- What are the current methods employed by individuals to dispose of unused and expired pharmaceuticals?
- Is their choice of disposal methods influenced by any prior knowledge of environmental issues associated with pharmaceuticals?
- Most importantly, is there a need for a formalized protocol for disposal and destruction of unused and expired medications worldwide in order to minimize their potential impact on the global environment?

1.6 Research Objectives

1. To review the policies adopted by the India and other countries towards use and disposal of medicines.

[2] https://www.ipc.gov.in/images/news/NFI-0414979118.pdf

[3] https://ipc.gov.in/mandates/nfi/release-of-national-formulary-of-india-2021.html

2. To find out the awareness and knowledge concerning the correct disposal of unused and expired drugs among student households in Gujarat
3. To find out the general practices concerning the correct disposal of unused and expired drugs among healthcare professionals
4. To suggest suitable policy measure for better awareness among the stakeholder concerning use of unused and disposal of date expired medicine.

1.7 Research Hypothesis

- H0 = There is no awareness among the students and households about disposal of medicines
- H1 = There is adequate awareness among the students and households about disposal of medicines

1.8 Data and Methodology

1.8.1 *Study Area*

The study was conducted in the state of Gujarat covering the respondents from rural, semi-urban and urban areas of Gujarat (Map 1.1)

Map 1.1: Location Map of Study Area

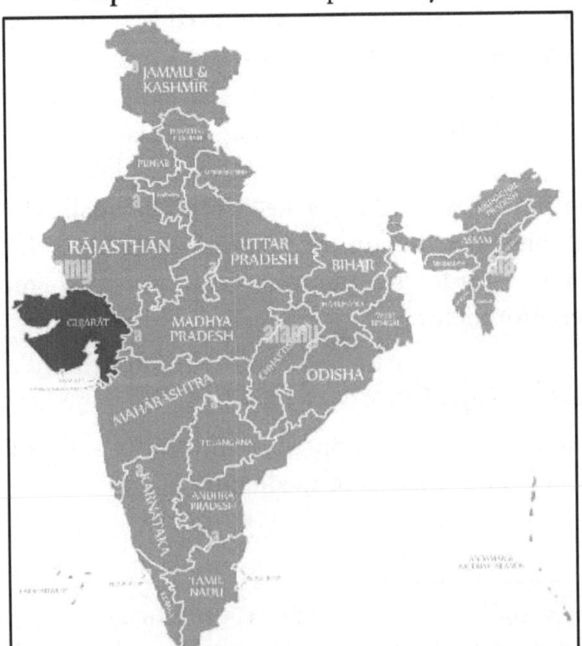

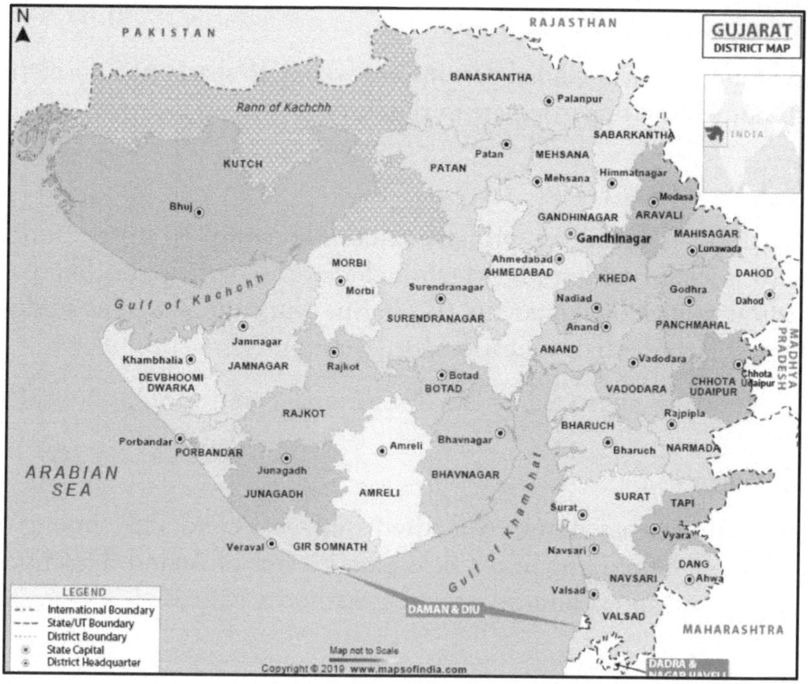

1.8.2 *Study Population*

Most of the healthcare professional was not aware of proper drug disposal and their impacts. Taken together, this study was planned to introduce healthcare professionals (student of pharmacy and students pursing nursing course) and students of Bachelor of education and other streams (trainee teachers) to assess their knowledge, practice and awareness towards safe disposal of expired drugs. Hence, the main objective of the study is to find out the knowledge, general practices, awareness, concerning the correct disposal of unused and expired drugs among healthcare professionals and student households in Gujarat. This study encompassed individuals of all genders aged 18 years and above, residing in the above-mentioned study area, with no specified upper age limit for inclusion in the study.

Inclusion criteria

The inclusion criteria for the study comprise individuals with exposure to medicines during the previous three months, who are willing to share information, with a minimum age requirement of 18 years. Additionally, registered pharmacies in Anand city are considered eligible participants.

Exclusion criteria

Exclusion criteria included persons not willing to share the information and not willing to participate in the study.

1.8.3 *Sources of Data*

The study is based on primary data. The study is cross-sectional, questionnaire-based study which included the participants like para-medical professional students (B Pharm, Nursing) as well as students of other faculties like education (Bed) and others.

The study was approved by the Institutional committee.

1.8.4 *Method*

Questionnaire-based, mixed-method study was conducted among the general public residing in the field practice area of Anand. Descriptive statistics and an exploratory research method are used.

1.8.5 *Sample Size*

The respondents were selected from three localities, viz. rural, semi-urban, and urban areas in Gujarat.

Assuming p=50% (50% of the general public lack proper knowledge regarding safe disposal of unused medicines) as previously no similar study had been conducted in this area. With absolute precision d=5% with a 95% confidence interval, we calculated the sample size to be 385 from the general public. A sample of 400 (385 respondents + 15 pharmacists) were selected. The respondents comprised group of students from:

- Pharmacy
- Nursing
- Bachelor of Education & Others

For the qualitative part, 15 registered pharmacists of the city located in and around the study area were also included in this study.

1.8.6 *Schedule/Questionnaire Development*

The questionnaire was developed in two languages-English and Gujarati and participants could choose either version based on their preference.

The questionnaire comprised two parts. The initial part focused on gathering personal details of the study participants, such as gender, age, marital status, education, occupation, and number of family members. The second part delved into the practices and perceptions of the respondents regarding the disposal of unused medication.

The questionnaire was pre-validated by doing a pilot study on 5 randomly selected participants. The questionnaire was modified based on the results obtained from the pilot study. Copy of final schedule is enclosed in annexure of this report.

1.8.7 *Data Collection*

All the participants were provided with the pre-validated self-administered questionnaire. Before filling out the questionnaire, the importance and purpose of the study were explained to the participants. After obtaining informed consent, the semi-structured schedules/questionnaires were canvassed/distributed to them, and sufficient time was given to the participants to fill out the questionnaire. For illiterate study participants, the interviewer read out the questionnaire and options before them and recorded their responses. For the registered pharmacies, a key informant interview was carried out among expert members regarding the disposal of expired medicines. The data were collected from July 2024 to October 2024.

1.8.8 *Analysis Techniques*

A simple tabular analysis was used. The data was analyzed with the help of descriptive statistics. Descriptive statistics was used to demonstrate the different variables. The quantitative data were computed as percentages and presented in tables.

1.9 Limitations

The study is based on the information provided by the respondents and thus accuracy of same depends on same.

1.10 Organisation of Book

The book is presented in five chapters. The introductory chapter presented in brief about the topic, method of disposal suggested by WHO need of the study, data and method used for the present study.

The second chapter present review of literature of past studies. Third chapter presented guidelines and policies towards disposal of medicine across globe. Next chapter presents the results of survey data and discussion on same. The last chapter present summary and conclusions.

The next chapter presents review of past studies.

CHAPTER II

Review of Literature

2.1 Introduction

The study objectives included reviewing procedures adopted by the general public for disposing of pharmaceuticals and public awareness about the problem of incorrect disposal methods. The literature search was done by searching related articles on websites and journal. The purpose of this systematic review was to determine the practice of medication disposal around the world and get insight into possible association between environmental awareness and people's behaviour regarding this issue.

2.2 Review of Literature

The review of literature is divided into four groups related to following aspects in order to understand the same.

1. Use of Medicine and its Storage
2. Disposal of Medicines
3. Impact on Environment
4. Policies and Programs

2.2.1 *Use of Medicine and its Storage*

Safe use of medicine includes safe storage and disposal. It is crucial that we organize and keep track of the drugs that we use. After all, you want to know where a particular medicine is when you or someone else needs it. There is a need to keep your drugs secure so that a curious toddler, a meddling teenager, a beloved pet or even houseguest, does not have access to the drugs easily. It have been also reported that some medicines are shared with friends and relatives. The re-use of leftover drugs for self-medication is unsafe which should be used only under the supervision of medical professional especially antibiotics and other prescription drugs. Expenditures for prescription and over-the-counter medications constitute a large percentage of total health care costs. High costs of medicines contribute to decrease in access to healthcare (Roy, *et al.*, 2012). Thus, unused or expired medications that are discarded represent a direct loss of revenue not only for the consumer alone, but also for pharmaceutical manufacturers, healthcare providers and ultimately to health of any nation.

Several factors, including the aging population, the prevalence of chronic diseases, and the growing number of treatments available, have contributed to an increase in medicine consumption and, consequently, the generation of pharmaceutical waste (OECD, 2021). Pharmaceutical waste refers to unnecessary medications that have expired or remain unused and are no longer needed (Chartier, 2014; West, 2015).

Abdi *et al.* (2011) noted that possibility of self-medication is higher in health sciences students than other students because of easy access to drug information resources and relatively sufficient familiarity with various kinds of drugs.

Gupta *et al.* (2018) studied awareness regarding disposal of unused medicines among consumers ar a tertiary care teaching hospital of North India and found that majority of participants 56.36% stated 1–5 drugs were left-over drugs at their homes. Most of the leftover medicines were analgesics in 59.1% followed by antibiotics in 51.36%. Most common dosage form of these leftover medicines were tablets in 85.9% of respondents. Majority of the respondents (55.9%) were not aware of the adverse outcomes of the pharmaceuticals in the environment.

Althagaf *et al.* (2022) assessed knowledge and awareness of safe disposal of unused or expired medication in Saudi Arabia and found that (49.1%) of participants stored medicines at home and these medicines were mainly stored in the refrigerator (64.4%). Non-prescribed medicines (67%) were mainly stored as unused or expiry medicines at home followed by prescribed medicines (51.9%). The main reason for the storage of unused/expired medicines at home was stopped medication after recovery (68.5%).

Shoaib *et al.* (2022) studied disposal practices of unused and expired pharmaceuticals among the general public in Quetta city, Pakistan found that improper storage and disposal of unused and expired medications is a common practice among study respondents in Pakistan and raised serious concerns.

Köksoy (2024) studied the unused, expired pharmaceuticals and their disposal practices among the general public in Burdur-Türkiye and found that there was a significant amount and number of unused medicines in households, and self-medication was common. Medicines were not properly disposed of and some of them had expired.

2.2.2 *Disposal of Medicines*

Drug disposal is the discarding of drugs. People generally dispose of unused drugs that remain after the end of medical treatment. Health care organizations dispose of drugs on a larger scale for a various reason, including having leftover drugs after treating patients and discarding of expired drugs. Failure to proper disposal of drugs creates opportunities for others (of whom the drug is unintended) to take them inappropriately. Inappropriate disposal of drugs can also cause drug pollution. People dispose of drugs in numerous ways. Even though organizations have expertise on drugs, they give inconsistent information about drug disposal to the consumers. Expired drugs should be disposed-off safely, without causing harm to the people and the environment. Unwanted & expired pharmaceuticals pose a higher risk to people, the environment, and wildlife (Daughton & Ternes, 1999; Vollmer, 2010; Zuccato *et al.*, 2004).

Improper medicine disposal poses environmental and public health risks, with common methods like flushing or throwing in the trash being detrimental. Proper disposal of pharmaceuticals should be well known among end-users. However, environmentally unsafe medication disposal practices are common in several regions of the world. For example, in Indonesia, it was found that >50% of the patients flushed their medicines down the toilet and <1% returned unused medication to the pharmacy (Insani *et al.*, 2020)˙ Other studies carried out in China (Wang *et al.*, 2016), India (Manocha, *et al.*, 2020) and Ghana (Sasu *et al.*, 2022) also found that the most common method of disposing of unused medication was throwing in the garbage, which ended up in landfills. These challenges and practice of improper pharmaceutical waste disposal has been well documented in review carried out among East African countries including Burundi, Kenya, Rwanda, South Sudan, Tanzania & Uganda despite the fact that there are measures for disposal in these countries. It has been discovered that the general public lacks sufficient understanding of how to dispose of unutilized, unneeded, and expired pharmaceuticals (Medhi & Sewal, 2012).

Abrous *et al.* (2010) studied safe medication disposal through student pharmacist and found that at baseline, 12.8% of patients disposed of medication appropriately. Respondents frequently flushed medications down the toilet (27.2%) or incorrectly dumped medications in the trash (34.6%). Only 30.9% had received previous advice on safe medication disposal.

Paut *et al.* (2016) found that the most common method for disposal of unused medications in households is disposal in the garbage (Kuwait, United Kingdom, Lithuania, Qatar, Serbia, Ghana, Bangladesh, Malta and Saudi Arabia). The practice of flushing drugs into the sewage system still takes place in New Zealand, USA and Bangladesh. Only in Sweden and Germany, practice of returning drugs to pharmacy was practiced to a larger extent. The environmental impact of improper medication disposal is expected in countries with poorly functioning waste management schemes (Middle Eastern, Asian and African countries).

Althagafia *et al.* (2022) assessed knowledge and awareness of safe disposal of unused or expired medication in Saudi Arabia and household trash was the most frequent method of disposal (79.5%). Author also found that only 8.4% of participants had received appropriate education or training related to the correct disposal of medication. The best-practiced method to increase community awareness regarding the disposal of unused or expiry medicine was awareness through social networking (70.3%). Authors suggested that patients' education regarding safe medication disposal and availability of medication disposal program.

Kamal *et al.* (2022) conducted study on disposal practices for unused and expired medications and found that majority of respondents in the three cities of the three countries expressed their interest in acquiring more knowledge on the recommended methods of medication disposal. Given the universal safety issue around inappropriate medication disposal, there is a need for counselling protocols regarding proper disposal, which can lead to better adherence, reduction of prescription drug abuse, and less environmental hazards due to prescription medications. The pilot study was able to identify population characteristics and logistical research issues in the three countries and will be vital in planning a proposed multi-country intervention on addressing people's behavior related to disposal of expired and unused medications.

Aryal *et al.* (2023) noted that medicines are crucial in treating various diseases, but when they are not needed, it is essential to dispose of them correctly. He noted that in many nations, disposing of unwanted drugs has become a burden since pharmaceutical waste permeates the ecosystem, posing a severe risk to human and environmental health. As a need of the hour, public education on proper medication disposal is required. Furthermore, the government should promote the reverse distribution practice. Residents are urged to return undesired prescriptions to pharmacies, which are collected and destroyed by approved agents or bodies.

Across Countries

Bound and Voulvoulis (2005) conducted a survey in the UK and revealed unhealthy practices of 400 households where they disposed unused and expired pharmaceuticals either as household waste or via the sink or toilet.

Ruhoy and Daughton (2005 & 2008) studied household disposal of pharmaceuticals as a pathway for aquatic contamination in the United Kingdom and noted that sink, toilet, and rubbish bins are the most commonly used but environmentally unfriendly routes of drug disposal. A huge pileup of expired and unused medications in the medicine cabinets among public reflects ignorance regarding disposal techniques.

A few studies have explored drug disposal practices in the United States[1]. A randomized controlled trial study showed that more than half of the patients (54%) had unused opioid analgesics after surgery and behavioral intervention such as directing patients to drug disposal programs, led to a 22% increase in the number of patients who reported disposing of or intending to dispose of their medications (Maughan, *et al.*, 2016). Yanovitzky (2016) reported that people exposed to media encouraging proper drug disposal practices were twice as likely to prefer appropriate disposal for their medications than those who were not exposed. A study conducted among university students by Matson (2015) showed that 77% of them did not store their medications in a locked or safe place and 28% of students witnessed sharing of prescription medications among peers.

---

[1] Kamal *et al.* (2022).

Another study by Lewis (2014) reported that 65.4% of patients surveyed keep and maintain their opioid medications even when not actively treating pain. An additional factor to consider is that patients improperly handle or share their medications due to possessing an excessive amount of medications. One study examined the extent, amount, type, cost, and reasons for unused medications in US households. Surveys administered at 20 drug disposal events showed that two-thirds of returned prescriptions (for tablet, capsule, and liquid dosage forms) had more than half the original quantity remaining [Law *et al.*, 2015]. The results showed that two-thirds of the returned medications were expired, 25% of them were discontinued by a physician, and 18% of them were discontinued by the patient once they were feeling better. It was also noted that 71% of patients chose a pharmacy as their preferred medication disposal location. These results are significant because excessive medication wastage is estimated to cost $2.4 billion among elderly populations and $5.4 billion among US adults [Law *et al.*, 2015]. In addition to the substantial economic impact, environmental concerns have also been raised concerning the improper disposal of unused and expired medications including the specific effects of antibiotics, estrogens and antidepressant medications upon wildlife and possible effects upon hu man health by continued exposure. A study conducted by the USFDA shows that between 2004 and 2014 there has been a 742%, 564%, and 122% increase in environmental concentrations of buprenorphine, naloxone, and naltrexone, respectively. These increases can be attributed to increased clinical use (Khan *et al.*, 2017). There is limited data on other medications being flushed and subsequently permeating the water supply. Despite the lack of studies on the topic, many counties across the US have "don't flush" programs. These programs encourage households to not introduce medications to the water supply in order to decrease water pollution [Sacramento Regional County Sanitation Department, 2019).

Kozak *et al.* (2016) studied need of assessment of unused and expired medication disposal practices in Indiana. The study was conducted by Medication Safety Research Network of Indiana covering 200 patients drawn from 15 different community pharmacies in Indiana that were part of a practice-based research network. Study found that although 40% of patients were conscious of the unused and expired medication take-back location in their community, only 15% adhered to it.

About 77% of patients were willing to adapt to a take-back location to return unused and expired medication. It was noted that the vulnerable populations lacked knowledge about unused and expired medication and access to proper disposal.

Vatovec *et al.* (2017) conducted a survey at the University of Vermont (US) to investigate the buying, usage, and disposal procedures among youths, the findings conveyed that 94% of the students had bought medicines in the early 12 months, 61% had 10 drugs leftover, and 18% of students had disposed of the drugs. The most common method of drug disposal was municipal trash (25%) and flushing (1%). Only 4% of the students used the drug take-back service and only 24% were conscious of drug take-back programs.

Ehrhart, *et al.* (2020) investigated pharmacist attitudes toward and recommendations about leftover drug disposal in United States and compared responses at locations with and without droboxes as well explored obstacles to drop box adoption and usage. Author found that customer awareness of drop boxes as well as knowledge about risks of improper disposal are low, however awareness was greater at pharmacies with drop boxes. Additionally, pharmacists at drop box locations were more consistent in their messaging to customers, more likely to recommend proper disposal methods, and more supportive of drug take-back programs. Through a focus group, we learned that further consumer education would overwhelm the capacity of the existing drop boxes. Based on our findings, authors recommend solutions to improper disposal focus on legislation mandating drop boxes at pharmacies and pressure on the pharmaceutical industry to fund proper disposal of unused pharmaceuticals.

African Countries

Sasu *et al.* (2012) conducted a study in Ghana about the disposal of unused and expired drugs at home and in hospitals. This study included five healthcare institutions, and general public involved 83 participants. The outcome of this study conveyed that among the five hospitals involved in the study, one quasi-governmental hospital has implemented a drug disposal program called the Disposal of Unused Medicines Program, and there are no separate drug disposal programs provided by the other hospitals. The general public polled that they admitted keeping unwanted or expired drugs at houses, and more than 75% said that they disposed of medicinal waste in regular trash cans, which ended up in landfills or disposal sites.

Auta *et al.* (2012) conducted survey among students of the pharmacy department at the University of Jos in Nigeria. This study showed the reasons for having pharmaceuticals in their homes were for emergency usage or comparable illnesses. The survey report emphasized that none of the survey participants returned unused medications to pharmacies. The majority of responses revealed that they threw away unwanted and expired prescriptions in garbage cans or dustbins. About 72.2% of respondents reported that they threw away their unneeded pills in the garbage.

Atinafu *et al.* (2015) conducted survey in Gondar, Ethiopia, regarding the unwanted drug disposal process showed that 89.1% had unused medications of which 57.3% of participants conveyed the reason for having unused drugs was due to a chronic disease condition. Also, the disposal methods preferred by the respondents were to keep the unutilized medications in their homes or throw them into the garbage or flush them into the toilet. The survey results also convey that about 75.3% of participants favored appropriate household World Health Organization (WHO) and U.S. Food and Drug Administration (FDA) drug disposal methods.

Wondimu *et al.* (2015) conducted study in the Tigray Region of Northern Ethiopia on drug storage and related issues disclosed that 29% of household participants had stored drugs and were not adequately identified. In contrast, according to 36% of respondents, the central place of drug storage was the drawer base cabinet. It also reported that most medications retained at home are not appropriately labeled or stored in a secure location. The presence of health professionals at home and in the residence area (rural versus urban) would help and influence improving household drug storage ().

Angienda and Bukachi (2016) studied households knowledge and perceptions on disposal practices of unused medicines in Kenya and found that households' knowledge on disposal practises of unused medicines is relatively weak attributed to by lack of public outreach and awareness campaign, laxity on the side of medical and healthcare professionals to provide disposal guidance at hospitals and pharmacies, unclear disposal instructions on medicines packages and negligence to read the disposal instructions.

Orok *et al.* (2023) assessed assessment of knowledge, awareness and disposal practices of unused and expired household medicines in the

Parker Corner Road Community in Liberia and found that 71% of the respondents in Liberia reported that they had not received any information on safe disposal practices while 64.2% admitted that they often did not read and follow and disposal instructions. The most popular disposal practices were disposal of the drugs along with household waste (61.1%) and ushing them down the toilets or sinks (25.3%). Majority of the respondents (82.1%) were aware of the environmental and human health effects arising from improper disposal of unused and expired medicines while 64.2% usually read medicine disposal instruction on the package. Only about 3% of them were aware of expired medication take-back system. 37% of respondents were aware that unused and expired medicines need to be disposed of safely while as much as 33.3% knew nothing about medication expiration date.

Asian Countries

Abahussain *et al.* (2006) surveyed 300 Kuwaiti patients to assess their attitudes and practices regarding the safe disposal of unutilized and unneeded medications. Almost half of the respondents obtained prescription medicines, and nearly all had unutilized and unnecessary medication at their homes. The most common reasons for having unutilized medications were found to be a change of prescription drugs by the physician and self-discontinuation. The standard disposal method adopted by the majority of respondents was throwing unutilized medicines in the garbage cans or flushing them into the toilet. About 54% of patients polled for the procedure, which included transporting drugs to pharmacies for safe disposal and beneficial effect).

Ali *et al.* (2010) conducted a cross-sectional survey-based study with a set of questionnaires among 481 female university students at University Sains Malaysia to assess the presence, perceptions, and behaviors of the female students regarding the storage of medicines and self-medication. The results shows that about 93.1% of total students claimed that they store pharmaceuticals in their rooms, 70.7% stopped using prescription medications without a doctor's consultation, and also self-medication was high among the study population.

Sharma *et al.* (2012) undertook cross-sectional survey was to ascertain the prevalence, attitude, and behavior toward the storage of medication and self-medication practices among young people in

Karnataka, India. Out of 150 respondents, 84.62% kept medications in their rooms. Self-medication was observed in 88.6% of people. The reasons for self-medication were a lack of knowledge about the disease condition and its treatment, the desire to save time, and the prescriber's ineffective medications.

Arkaravichien *et al.* (2014) studied environmental impact of drug disposal practices in Thailand, the most typical disposal method was discarding medicines in a trash bin. It involved the participation of 331 people in the survey with questions about how medications are stored, the storage procedure, and their management of leftover medications. The study showed that about 89.4% of people retained leftover medications at home and threw away the medicines when no longer needed. Trashing into a garbage bin was the most common practice for disposing of medicine. Disposed drugs were 81.4% of solid dosage form, 64.6% of liquid dosage form, and 66.6% of drugs used for external application. About 7.4% of respondents conveyed that drugs belonging to liquid formulations were disposed of into the drainage system).

Al-Shareef *et al.* (2016) conducted a cross-sectional study and investigated participants' attitudes toward disposing of unutilized and expired medications conducted in Riyadh, Saudi Arabia. About 1,200 patients were randomly chosen from King Khalid University Hospital and King Saud University. Participants were asked to fill out a paper- based questionnaire that included self-enumeration. A significant proportion of respondents disposed of unutilized medications through household waste, while a small proportion of about 1.7% returned those medications to a pharmacy.

Pankajkumar *et al.* (2016) conducted observational, prospective self-administered cross- sectional study with a sample size of 372 participants to study the storage and disposal practice of medicines at home among pharmacy, nursing, and arts and science students in Gandhinagar, Gujarat, India. The survey was conducted in pre- and post-education sessions using a predefined questionnaire. According to the findings of this study, respondents threw their unwanted or expired medications in the trash bins. The study also concluded that students' knowledge of drug storage and disposal was insufficient and drug-use assessments were required to raise awareness about drug storage and disposal methods.

Labu and Harun-or-Rashid, (2016) conducted study in Bangladesh to assess safe disposal practices, 36.3% of the 290 students surveyed were aware of the term "medication trash." The majority of participants reported that drugs belonging to liquid and solid dosage forms were disposed of and ended up in a landfill. About 73% of them said that solid dosage form is disposed of in landfills. According to the findings of this survey, there seems to be an urgent need to raise public awareness and develop dispensing guidelines that reduce the volume of medication waste.

Bashaar *et al.* (2017) conducted a cross-sectional survey study in Kabul, Afghanistan, aimed to demonstrate the disposal practices of the general public for unused drugs in Kabul. It involved 301 respondents directly interviewed for questionnaires regarding disposal practices among the general public. The study results conveyed that about 95.3% kept their medications at home, and 77.7% of participants responded that expired medications were disposed of in trash cans at home. A proportion of participants claimed that the government should be responsible for increasing public awareness about proper medicine disposal. Most respondents agreed that improper management of unoccupied and expired medications might influence human health and the environment

Gupta *et al.* (2013) studied patient's opinion and practice towards unused medication disposal and found that most common method followed by majority of the participants for disposing of the solid, semi-solid and liquid dosage forms was garbage in 95%, 91.4% and 76.4% of consumers respectively. About 9.31% of the participants were in favour of initiating a program to collect unused medications from home.

Gupta *et al.* (2018) investigated awareness regarding disposal of unused medicines among consumers ar a tertiary care teaching hospital of North India found that majority of participants 56.36% stated 1–5 drugs were left-over drugs at their homes. Most of the leftover medicines were analgesics in 59.1% followed by antibiotics in 51.36%. Most common dosage form of these leftover medicines were tablets in 85.9% of respondents. Majority of the respondents (55.9%) were not aware of the adverse outcomes of the pharmaceuticals in the environment. The most common method followed by majority of the participants for disposing of the solid, semi-solid and liquid dosage forms was garbage in 95%, 91.4% and 76.4% of consumers respectively. About 9.31% of the participants were in favour of initiating a program to collect unused medications from home.

Raja *et al.* (2018) investigated awareness and disposal practices of unused and expired medication among health care professionals and students in a tertiary care teaching hospital found that the commonest discarding pattern of the expired/ unused medicines was through household trash (67%). A total of 349 (89%) were aware of the significance of improper disposal. It was observed that the participants 44 (11.1%) had partial knowledge about proper drug disposal but there was a lack of practice (67.1%) of safe disposal methods. About 264(17%) participants mentioned that by throwing in thrash is the major route of drug disposal followed by crushing the drugs before discarding (17%), flushing in toilets or sinks (6%) and only 5% return the drugs to the medical store.

Alhomoud *et al.* (2020) conducted study in Saudi Arabia and found that majority of students (79%) stored their medication in a bedroom or kitchen. Gender-specific variables revealed a gender difference in storing and disposing of these medications. Many students reported previously discarding medicines in the garbage (89%) or giving them to someone else to use (22%). More than half of the sample (60%) had not received any information on how to store or dispose of medications.

Alshehri and Banjar (2021) studied increasing awareness of proper disposal of unused and expired medication using a knowledge-based disposal management system and found that 66.8% of the 310 participants had unneeded medications in their homes, and only 14.9% knew how to dispose of unusable medications, while only 6.5% knew how to dispose of expired medications. Overall, the research studied Saudi society's behaviour regarding unused and expired medications, and created a prototype of a knowledge-based system designed to increase awareness of proper disposal and management of unused and expired medications.

Bashatah and Wajid (2021) investigated the knowledge and practices concerning unused and expired medicine among pharmacy and nursing students at King Saud University, Riyadh, Saudi Arabia. The study results indicated that 57.4% of pharmacy students and 53.4% of nursing students check the expiry date of medicine before procuring, and 37.6% of pharmacy students and 52.5% of nursing students keep unused medicine until it expires. With regard to disposal, 78.9% of pharmacy students and 80.5% of nursing students reported discarding expired medicine in household garbage or flushing it down a sink or toilet. Only a small percentage returns leftover medicine to a medical store.

Begum *et al.* (2021) investigated disposal practises in Dhaka and findings disclose that, for most of the key informants, the terms "drug disposal" and "drug pollution" were unknown; more precisely, 67% and 74% of key informants even did not hear these two terms. Almost all (87%) households faced undesired incidents due to the insecure storage of medicines. People disposed of excess and expired medication in regular dustbins (47%), threw out of the window (19%), flushed within commode (4%), burnt in fire (2%), and reused (4%). A good percentage of people (21%) returned unexpired drugs to the pharmacy and bought other medicines on a need basis. A total of 72% wanted a medicine take-back program, and 100% agreed on mass education on this issue.

Alghadeer and Al-Arifi (2021) conducted study in Saudi Arabia and found that more than 70% returned the unused drugs to the pharmaceutical distributors. Around 80% of the participants confirmed the risk of environmental damage due to the inappropriate disposal of drugs, and 87.5% of them held themselves responsible for preventing such risk. Approximately 85% of surveyed pharmacists believed community pharmacies to be an appropriate location for the collection of unused drugs.

Jha *et al.* (2022) conducted study in Nepal and found that nearly 90% of respondents agreed that storage of excess medicines at home may promote self-medication. Similarly, 97.6% of respondents agreed there is a lack of adequate information on the safe disposal of unused medicines. The majority [125 (59.5%)] of participants always checked the expiry date of medicines. The safe methods of medicine disposal were not known by 137 (65.2%) participants. Throwing in a dustbin was the preferred method of expired medicine disposal.

Kanyari *et al.* (2024) studied disposal practices of unused and expired medicines among the general public and pharmacies: a mixed-method study in the Odisha State of Eastern India and found that 97.4% disposed of unused drugs improperly, whereas only 2.6% returned the expired drugs to the pharmacy. Improper disposal of unused and expired medicines is becoming a global problem, especially in developing countries such as India. It is much more because of poor regulation of the health sector, and a significant part of the population is less aware of the drug disposal policies and hazards associated with their improper implementation. Addressing the issue of unused and expired medicines in India requires a multifaceted approach involving individuals, healthcare providers, pharmaceutical companies, and government bodies to ensure efficient resource utilization, reduce waste, and safeguard public health and the environment.

European Countries

Coma *et al.* (2008) conducted survey to carry out in community pharmacies in Barcelona, Spain, to investigate the number of unutilized drugs and their cost to the public health system. According to the findings, approximately 52.4% handed back their prescription in person, while 32.2% handed back by their relative. The reason behind returning medications was the expiry date. About 24.9% of patients conveyed that the drugs were no longer required as their health conditions improved. This study emphasized the significance of returning unutilized medicines that would reduce unnecessary health expenditure. It also marked the shortcomings of the Spanish healthcare system in terms of prescription, dispensing procedures, and the use of medications.

Vellinga *et al.* (2014) conducted a survey of 398 randomly selected people in Ireland to analyze baseline knowledge on medicine storage and disposal among the general public. About 88% of respondents reported that they retain unutilized medications at home, and the common reason conveyed by 68% of respondents for storing unutilized medications was to keep them for later use. The sewage system and general waste disposal used by the study respondents were both environmentally unsound methods. Surprisingly, 75% of people who had received advice on proper disposal practices from a healthcare professional disposed of their medicine correctly.

Bungau *et al.* (2018) conducted a survey of Romanian pharmacists about unused and expired medicines and analyzed the factors that may affect the efficiency of pharmacies in collecting and disposing of the medications used by the population. This survey included 521 pharmacists of which 16% of them worked in pharmacies that did not allow the process of collecting unutilized or expired drugs from the community, and 33% of pharmacies refused to take unutilized medicines from the general public at least once. The most common reasons given by pharmacists for refusing to collect back the unutilized medications included the lack of procedure, insufficient legislation, exceeding the amount contracted with the operators, and high costs.

Map 2.1: Methods of Drug Disposal and Frequencies in which they are Reported in Different Countries

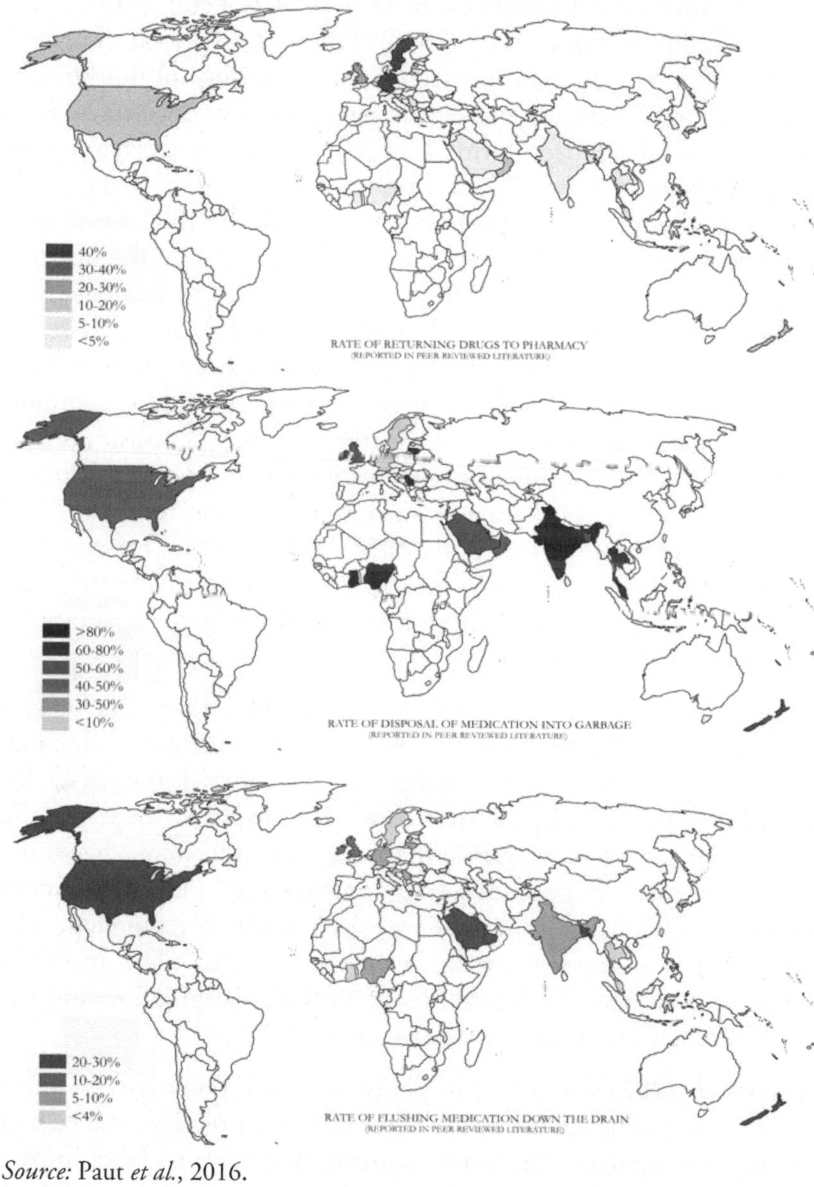

Source: Paut *et al.*, 2016.

2.2.3 *Impact on Environment*

The Pharmaceuticals have been detected throughout the environment where at least in some cases, they have been shown to have a detrimental effect. Many results from improper patient disposal of unused pharmaceuticals via environmentally-unfriendly routes, such as the sink, toilet or rubbish bin (Tong *et al.*, 2011). Pharmaceuticals may enter the environment through improper disposal of unused and expired pharmaceutical dosage forms in the toilet or sink (Ruhoy and Daughton, 2007, Comeau *et al.*, 2008). Processes employed in sewage treatment plants are often ineffective in removing all improperly disposed pharmaceuticals and therapeutic medication excreted in unchanged or metabolized forms from effluent before discharge into waterways (Nakada *et al.*, 2006, Kim and Aga, 2007, Zorita *et al.*, 2009) and thus pharmaceuticals can potentially be discharged into waterways. If unwanted pharmaceuticals are disposed of in the garbage, they eventually end up in landfills with the potential to be discharged into the environment as leachate (Barnes *et al.*, 2004). Some classes of returned medicines go through incineration, which depends on each country's regulation. However, open burning is still a common practice, mainly in developing countries, where the waste is not separate at all. Open burning of healthcare waste is a potential source of carbon and other contaminants such as dioxins and furans (WHO 1999; Babanyara *et al.*, 2013; Raila 2017). Black carbon, for example, may intensify global warming due to its capacity to absorb solar energy and increase dark cloud formation, decreasing its ability to reflect sunlight (DeAngelis 2011).

Pollution has been a challenge for sustainable development and pharmaceutical pollution has direct implications in the environmental, economic and social spheres, which are considered the triad for sustainable development. Drugs are designed to cause-specific biological effects at low concentrations and, therefore, have the potential to cause huge damage to organisms in the environment (Arnold *et al.*, 2014). To achieve sustainable development, the pharmaceutical residues must be properly managed. The incorrect disposal of pharmaceuticals involves decentralized legislation and the lack of information by society (Santos *et al.*, 2010).

Souza *et al.* (2021) noted that pharmaceutical pollution is still a problem, and going against SDGs from this point of view; the lack of drug disposal regulation in some countries may have a global impact and harm many ecosystems worldwide; the solutions indicated here would integrate the management and help to reduce drug pollution, consequently, moving towards SGDs.

2.2.4 *Awareness, Policies and Steps*

While it is clear that environmental awareness may impact the choice of what is considered the safest mean of disposal, actual behavior does not always equate the awareness. However, this gap between the possession of environmental knowledge and awareness, and displaying pro-environmental behavior is well known. For decades, researchers have sought to understand and map the factors that lead people to delay or to fail to move from environmental knowledge to pro-environmental behavior. An individual's perception of the extent to which his or hers actions can truly help to improve the environment and sense of personal responsibility can both contribute to people's behavior (Gifford and Nilsson 2014).

Aditya (2013) recommended the need to improve their awareness about safe and prudent disposal methods through sensitization of undergraduate students.

Paut *et al.* (2016) found that lack of the adequate information and clear instructions on proper manners of drug disposal was reported in many surveyed countries (USA, New Zealand, Bangladesh, Malta and Ireland). Clear and definite connection between knowledge about environmental detrimental effects of improper drug disposal and the preference towards disposal methods could not be established. Many respondents were generally concerned with issues of inadequate medicines discarding but the behavior regarding disposal of unused drugs often did not equate the awareness (Serbia, USA, Kuwait, Malta and UK). The current data emphasizes the global issue of improper medicine disposal, prevalent in environmentally-aware people.

Klatte *et al.* (2017) summarized some measures to reduce pharmaceuticals in the environment. First of all, it is necessary to review the entire process, from the pharmaceutical production to the prescribers, the consumer, and the final destination, rather than only the final disposal as considered in many national regulations. It is required that doctors and health professionals understand the issue and guide the patients into conscious consumption. Moreover, effluent monitoring, whether industrial or domestic is essential to ensure that they are free of pharmaceutical residues.

Shivaraju and Gangadhar (2017) studied knowledge and awareness of disposal of unused and expired medications among medical undergraduates of a tertiary care teaching hospital at B G Nagar in Karnataka and found that awareness of proper and safe drug disposal among the medical students was quite fair and suggested to implement educational programs regularly.

Manocha *et al.* (2020) studied current disposal practices of unused and expired medicines among general public in Delhi and national capital region, India and found that majority (93%) of consumers were in favour of a government program to collect unused or expired medicines from their home. Authors suggested that the knowledge and practices of consumers towards disposal of unused and expired medicines needs to be improved. Health care professionals, government and policy makers should offer training to educate and guide the general public on safe and proper disposal practices of expired or unused medicines.

Chaturvedi *et al.* (2021) noted that as per published literature reports, the removal of antibiotics and related traces being difficult, couples the possibility of emergence of antibiotic resistance and hence sustainability in global water resources. Therefore, research on environmental behavior and control strategies should be conducted along with assessing their chronic toxicity to identify potential human and ecological risks.

Toe *et al.* (2023) observed that around 71% of the respondents reported that they had not received any information on safe disposal practices while 64.2% admitted that they often did not read and follow disposal instructions. The most popular disposal practices were disposal of the drugs along with household waste (61.1%) and flushing them down the toilets or sinks (25.3%). Majority of the respondents (82.1%) were aware of the health effects arising from improper disposal of unused and expired medicines while 64.2% usually read medicine disposal instruction on the package. Only about 3% of them knew of expired medication take-back system and 33.3% knew nothing about medication expiration date. The study revealed insufficient knowledge as well as inappropriate disposal practices of unused and expired medicines among residents of Parker Corner Road Community in Brewerville. There is need to organize a public enlightenment programme on safe, appropriate use, as well as disposal of unused and expired medicines.

Many technological initiatives have been adopted worldwide to reduce pharmaceutical pollution, but some simpler initiatives, such as campaigns for the correct disposal of medicines or avoiding polypharmacy in older people, may be very effective in minimizing the risks. It is suggested a global cooperation sharing investment in research to a better understanding of pharmaceuticals in the environment and share technologies. Therefore, an international agreement for the reduction and mitigation of pharmaceutical pollution would benefit the entire population, while the lack of it is generating cascading effects reaching human and environmental health.

Since drugs are not entirely removed in water and sewage treatment plants nowadays, it is crucial to support new technologies to remove these substances. The recent reviews by Kanakaraju *et al.* (2018), Mansour *et al.* (2018) and Rosman *et al.* (2018) describe drug removal technologies, mainly focusing on adsorption on activated carbons and advanced oxidation processes that employ ozone, ultraviolet radiation, gamma radiation and electro-oxidation. Some methods contemplated by those reviews present a removal potential up to 100% for some drugs. Although these techniques require a high operational cost, some countries already use them, such as Germany, Switzerland, and Sweden (Baresel *et al.*, 2019). The support for these technologies must be political since they have a significant social impact. However, the issue is more critical in developing countries since the sewage sometimes is not even collected, then it is also not treated at all.

2.3 Summary

Reviews of disposal practices for unused medications in India indicate that the most common method is simply throwing them in household garbage, with a significant portion of people also flushing them down the toilet, highlighting a lack of awareness and proper disposal systems for expired or unwanted medicines; most people would prefer to return unused medications to pharmacies if given the option, but access to such take-back programs is limited. The guidelines for disposal for medicines are prescribed by World Health Organization (WHO) and United States Food and Drugs Administration (USFDA). Some of the methods suggested to dispose date expired and unused medicines include returning to manufacturer, landfill, and waste immobilization: encapsulation/incertization, flushing it down the

Sewer and incineration. Despite precautions associated with these methods, these methods are not effective.

The next chapter presents guidelines and policies adopted by different countries towards disposal of medicine.

CHAPTER III

Guidelines and Policies towards Disposal of Medicines across Globe[1]

3.1 Introduction

Drug disposal practices vary widely globally due to many reasons; most of them are due to government regulations (Brechtelsbauer & Shah, 2020; Alnahas,2020; Hoque and Rafi, 2023; Freitas & Radis-Baptista, 2021], individual cultural attitudes (Ayele & Mamu, 2018; Angi'enda and Bukachi, 2016; Kampamba,2024; Kamal, 2022; Aditya & Singh, 2013; and Watkins, 2022), infrastructure of the healthcare system [de Campos EAR *et al.,* 2021; Kongar, 2015; Nyaga 2020; Mwita 2024; Daughton 2003), and last but not the least public awareness [Hoque and Rafi, 2023; Alghadeer & Al-Arifi 2021; Alshehri & Banjar 2022). These factors can affect drug disposal methods in different countries including South and South Asian regions. Understanding these factors helps to appreciate why drug disposal practices are so varied around the world and highlights the importance of context when addressing pharmaceutical waste management (Shwetha & Jha 2018; Raja *et al.,* 2018; and Tegegne *et al.,* 2024) (Uddin, *et al.*, 2024).

In the last decade, the disposal of unused or expired pharmaceuticals has gained a particular interest. The global increase in pharmaceutical spending has led to an enhanced international awareness on the issue of unused medications and harmful economic, environmental and health effects of improper medicine disposal (Braund *et al.,* 2009; EEA 2010; Kummerer 2008). Apart from the measures employed to reduce the creation of unused medication and lower the economic burden arising from direct costs of discarded medications (Ruhoy and Daughton 2007), country-wide plans for promoting and implementing adequate disposal methods can limit potentially damaging environmental effects (West *et al.,* 2014). The policies adopted by the

[1] This chapter heavily based on published paper and reviews. Corresponding references are cited and acknowledged.

some selected countries are presented and discussed below (based on published literature).

3.2 Brief Information on Regulations across Countries

As mentioned, and exemplified in the previous topic, pharmaceutical pollution is not in line with the SDGs. To achieve sustainable development, the pharmaceutical residues must be properly managed. The incorrect disposal of pharmaceuticals involves decentralized legislation and the lack of information by society (Santos *et al.*, 2010). Therefore, we reviewed the national laws present in the countries with the highest drug market according to Glassmeyer *et al.* (2009).

It was not long after pharmaceutical products became widely available in the 1940s that concerns over drug safety emerged, first in relation to human health (patient safety) and subsequently, to ecological health (environmental pollution) Daughton, CG (2016). In 1963, the World Health Assembly passed a resolution inviting its member States to systematically collect data on the serious adverse effects of drugs observed during drug development and after market entry (WHO, 1963). While formal frameworks for pharmacovigilance, i.e., drug safety, that were subsequently developed pertained exclusively to patient health, by the 1990s, it became widely recognized that pharmaceuticals are present in the environment and cause deleterious effects on the organisms exposed to them. There are three main pathways how pharmaceuticals reach the environment: (i) wastewater discharged from manufacturing facilities, (ii) normal consumer or animal use and (iii) improper disposal of unused or expired medicines by consumers.

The guidelines for disposal for medicines are prescribed by World Health Organization (WHO) and United States Food and Drugs Administration (USFDA). Some of the methods suggested to dispose date expired and unused medicines include returning to manufacturer, landfill, and waste immobilization: encapsulation/ inertization, flushing it down the Sewer and incineration. Despite precautions associated with these methods, these methods are not effective. Studies have shown that these methods sometime pose a risk not only to human beings by increasing chances of taking wrong medications, accidental poisoning, adverse drug reactions, drug-drug interactions that increases health burden but also to the environment. In India, the knowledge regarding disposal of date expired and unused medicines is lacking among common people.

Argentina establishes medicines return by the national decree n° 1.299/97 and the resolution 522/2016 provides measures for the correct management of household medicines referred as "Residues of special generation". The National Medicines Policy is an effective program for optimizing drug use in the Argentine health system, which is a real intervention from the government to bring information to the health system and patients (Cangenova 2006).

In South Australia, the disposal of medical waste is controlled by the Environment Protection Policy (Environment Protection Act, 1993), ensuring that people who generate medical waste should not cause environmental or human harm. Also, such waste should not be placed in the domestic collection service (EPA, 2003). Because that policy is not for the whole country, the Australian Government (Department of Health) funded the "Return Unwanted Medicines Project" in 1998, which is a national community pharmacy network aimed to collect unwanted or overdue drugs (Glassmeyer *et al.*, 2009; Wheeler 2017). After collection, the drugs are sent to the Environmental Protection Authority and incinerated at high temperatures for elimination (Murdoch 2015).

Brazil approved decree n° 10.388/2020, which includes medicines and their packages for human use, expired or in disuse in the reverse logistics system. In the Decree, the manufacturers, importers, distributors, traders, and consumers are responsible for implementing. It will initially include states and municipalities with a population greater than 500.000 inhabitants and, later, municipalities with a population greater than 100.000 inhabitants. Some municipalities already had legislation for the correct disposal of medicines by consumers (*e.g.,* Law n° 13.442/2016; Law n° 17.211/2012; Law n° 13.905/2012). About the drug disposal program, Brazil does not have any national coverage. However, some initiatives, such as the conscious disposal program, have collection points in some Brazilian states (Descarte Consciente, 2021).

Canada has no national provision program for the public in Canada. There is the Ontario Regulation n° 298/12, where producers must collect and dispose of pharmaceuticals brought by consumers, as well as the collection, recycling and/or disposal of their packages (Regulation n° 298/12, 1990). There are a variety of programs established at the provincial, municipal, and community level (Gagnon 2009). For example, in Alberta, pharmacies receive correct disposal instructions through the (Return Old or Unused Medications for Environmentally Friendly Disposal, 2021: https://rxa.ca/member-benefits/envirx/) program. This program is funded by the Alberta Pharmacists' Association, with donations from Innovative Medicines Canada and the Health Products Stewardship Association (Alberta Pharmacists' Association, 2021). The "Medications Return Program" of the British Columbia province dedicates efforts to collect unused or expired medicines from people before going to the garbage. They receive all prescription drugs, over-the-counter medicines, and natural health products. Health Products Stewardship Association manages the "Medications Return Program" since 1999 and is an initiative regulated explicitly in the Recycling Regulation (Regulation n°449/2004, Gagnon 2009).

In 2006, the Planning Conference and Resource Saving & Waste Management Groups collaborated with the Federation of Pharmaceutical Manufacturers Associations of Japan (FPMAJ) to promote solid waste disposal in the pharmaceutical industry (Hanashi 2011). In 2008, the Academic Committee of the Japan Hospital Pharmacist Association and the Environmental Safety Committee of the Association of Pharmaceutical Manufacturers of Japan released a document with guidelines for disposing of hospital waste (Pharmaceutical Packaging and Container Disposal Guide, 2007), especially pharmaceutical containers and packages. These products must be incinerated if the pharmaceutical products are inside the package and recycled or disposed of the empty ones. According to Glassmeyer *et al.* (2009), Japan ranks second among twelve nations in the pharmaceutical market. Consumers in Japan are advised to dispose of medical waste, including pharmaceuticals, in their household garbage (JPMA 2007). In 2014, Sanofi Company started the first program for the disposal of unused or expired medicines for members and 60% of employees participated in the first year (Sanofi, 2017).

The General Law for prevention and integral management of residues in Mexico as well as the general health law establishes the producers' responsibility of proper disposal of the waste generated to ensure environmental protection (Gracia-Vásquez *et al.*, 2015; Guzmán *et al.*, 2019; General Law, 2015; General Law 2021). The Official Mexican Standard (NOM-052-SEMARNAT, 2005) establishes the characteristics, the identification procedure, classification and the list of dangerous waste, including residues from pharmaceutical chemistry. Mexico has a national plan led by the health sector and pharmacy industry, where they are responsible for the management of expired medicines in the entire commercial chain (COFEPRIS, 2012; Jáuregui-Medina *et al.*, 2015). The National Management System of Residues of Medicines and Packages has collectors for medicines disposal covering 72% of the country's states (Jáuregui-Medina *et al.*, 2015; Singrem, 2021).

Although the Medicines Regulations 1984 (Regulations n°143/1984, updated in 2020) established that the General Director might request the destruction of medicines for any manufacturer or drugstore, there is no national policy for medicines disposal in New Zealand (Tong *et al.*, 2011a; Bisset, 2019). However, the country has the Disposal of Unwanted Medicines Properly Project (2020), encouraging society to return the medicines for the pharmacies. Moreover, the country also holds a program to distribute medicines for people who needs them worldwide by showing a prescription (Medical Aid Abrod, 2021). Although country has many programs for medicines disposal and distribution, a wide-range policy would help create public awareness and avoid environmental issues (Murdoch 2015).

The disposal of pharmaceuticals in the United States is regulated by Environmental Protection Agency (EPA), Drug Enforcement Administration (DEA) and Occupational Safety and Health Administration (OSHA) (Brechtelsbauer and Shah 2020). In 2019, the EPA published the Final Rule of Management Standards for Hazardous Waste Pharmaceuticals intended to change the Resource Conservation and Recovery Act (RCRA) regulation of hazardous waste pharmaceuticals (United States Environmental Protection Agency, 2019; Brechtelsbauer and Shah 2020). One aim is to avoid the pharmaceutical residues to reach the wastewater effluents due to the old practice of discarding medicines in the toilet (United States Environmental Protection Agency, 2019; Brechtelsbauer and Shah 2020). All the states have until July 2021 to adopt the final rule. All healthcare facilities and all reverse distributors should comply with the new rule managing all kinds of pharmaceuticals, except for small establishments with conditional exemption (United States Environmental Protection Agency, 2019; Brechtelsbauer and Shah 2020). The new EPA rule set the sewer prohibition, where pharmaceuticals may not be discarded in drain or toilet. However, the new rule did not include household generation of pharmaceutical waste, maintaining the take back programs and events managed by each state (US Environmental Protection Agency, 2019; Brechtelsbauer and Shah 2020).

Disposal of medical products in the United Kingdom is covered by Controlled Waste Regulation (1992) (HMSO, 1992), and clinical waste is controlled by Special Waste Regulation (1996) (HMSO, 1996; Bound and Voulvoulis 2005). According to this Law, such waste can be disposed of in landfills specifically designed for this type of waste or may be incinerated. The country also has an Action Plan elaborate in 2012 to minimize waste and improve drug use, such as encouraging the society to return medicines in pharmacies rather than stocking them (Government of United kingdom, 2012). Besides, the country also has pharmaceutical collection events held by National Health Service (NHS) (Kusturica *et al.*, 2016).

Pharmacies in the United Kingdom are obliged to take back unwanted and unused medicines brought by patients and return these to the NHS. The system only covers household waste and the local authorities are responsible for the final disposal and promote awareness campaigns (Health Care Without Harm 2013). The campaign encourages people to request only the pharmaceuticals that will be used to avoid waste generation (Medicine Waste UK, 2021: http://www.medicinewaste.com/campaign). In the United Kingdom, pharmacies and veterinary clinics can denature pharmaceutical residues according to their classification before disposal (UK Guidance, 2021).

The member states of the European Union shall ensure appropriate collection systems for medical products that are unused or have expired (Directive 2004/27/EC). The European Union also has some strategies for handling pharmaceutical pollution, such as understanding the pharmaceutical fate in the environment, awareness of rational use and support the development of less environmentally harmful pharmaceuticals (European Comission, 2019).

In France, Decree n° 92-377 had designated the packers' responsibility for the disposal of packaging waste. The French Law n° 248/2007 established that the pharmacies must receive unused pharmaceuticals (Law n° 248/2007). Moreover, France operates a structured industry-funded system for recalling pharmaceutical waste (Macarthur *et al.*, 2000; Defarges 2020). The collaborative system includes manufacturers, wholesalers and community pharmacies carried out by Cyclamed (Macarthur *et al.*, 2000). Cyclamed has contributed to the reduction of unused pharmaceuticals in France (Defarges 2020).

Updated in 2012, the German Waste Management Act established prevention and recycling to mitigate the waste impacts on the environment and human health (Germany Federal Environmental Agency, 2014). Although there is no specific regulation for medicine disposal, according to the Germany Federal Environmental Agency, pharmaceutical products can be disposed of in collection points or ordinary garbage since most of the waste is incinerated in the country Arzneimittel-Entsorgung richtig gemacht, 2021).

In Italy, decree n° 254/2003 encourages the authorities to reduce, recycle and, whenever possible, recover waste at the final destination. The Associazione Indennizzo Resi (Assinde) is responsible for managing the collection of unused drugs (Costa *et al.*, 2018). In the country, unused drugs are received in specific collectors in pharmacies, health centers, streets, and collection sites, depending on the municipality (Health Care Without Harm 2013). Municipalities can rely on public or private partnerships to manage and pay the costs involved in collecting and disposing of medicines. Italy was one of the first European countries to present a collection and disposal of drugs in the late 70's (Hiratuka *et al.*, 2013).

In Spain, Royal Decree n° 1345/2007 establishes the pharmaceutical sellers' responsibility to collect drugs from the household. Law n° 29/2006 determines that the medicine packages have the authorization symbol of the Spanish Agency for medicines and health products to assist the collection process. Spain also has Law n° 22/2011 - the general Law on solid waste and contaminated soils -, where the authorities do waste disposal in a way that does not impact the environment and public health. The country has a reverse logistics program for medicines (Bellan *et al.*, 2012). In 2002, the Integrated waste packaging management system was established by the Spanish National Association of the Pharmaceutical Industry, according to the Directive 94/62/CEE based on the expanded responsibility for medicine disposal management (Directive 94/62/CEE; Hiratuka *et al.*, 2013). The system collects unused, overdue, and even empty boxes of medicines (Coma *et al.*, 2008, SIGRE, 2021). The country also has awareness campaigns (Medsdisposal) to inform society about the correct disposal of drugs that involves some countries in Europe (MedsDisposal, 2021).

In India, drug regulation and control are primarily handled by the Central Drugs Standard Control Organization (CDSCO) under the Ministry of Health & Family Welfare, with the Drug Controller General of India (DCGI) as its head. Here's a more detailed breakdown:

Central Drugs Standard Control Organization (CDSCO):

- Is the national regulatory authority for drugs, pharmaceuticals, and medical devices in India.
- Responsible for approving new drugs, conducting clinical trials, setting drug standards, controlling the quality of imported drugs, and coordinating activities of state drug control organizations.
- The CDSCO also grants licenses for certain specialized categories of critical drugs.

Drug Controller General of India (DCGI):

- Is the head of the CDSCO.
- Responsible for approving licenses for specified categories of drugs, such as blood and blood products, IV fluids, vaccines, and sera.
- Also sets standards for manufacturing, sales, import, and distribution of drugs in India.

Narcotics Control Bureau (NCB):

- Is the nodal agency for drug law enforcement in India, focusing on preventing and combating drug abuse and illicit trafficking.

State Drug Control Organizations:

- Primarily responsible for the regulation of manufacture, sale, and distribution of drugs within their respective states.

Drugs & Cosmetic Act and Rules (DCA):

- The manufacturing, import, sale, and distribution of drugs are regulated under the DCA.

Ministry of Health & Family Welfare:

- The CDSCO functions under the Directorate General of Health Services, which falls under the Ministry of Health & Family Welfare.

National Formulary of India (NFI)

The 6th edition of the National Formulary of India, 2021 (NFI 2021) has been released on 28.10.2021 by Dr. Mansukh Mandaviya, Hon'ble Union Minister of Health & Family Welfare, Government of India along with officials of Ministry of Health & Family Welfare and IPC at Ministry of Health & Family Welfare, Nirman Bhawan, New Delhi. The principal objective of NFI is to promote rational use of medicines.

The National Formulary of India is essentially meant for the guidance of the members of the medical and pharmaceutical profession; medical students, nurses and pharmacists etc. working in hospitals, dispensaries and in sales establishments. In the preparation of this Formulary, the expert opinion of medical practitioners, teachers in medicine, nurses, pharmacists etc. has been obtained. The selection of drugs for inclusion in the National Formulary has been made taking into consideration the relative advantages and disadvantages of the various drugs used in current medical practice and their availability in the country. Thus the National Formulary of India represents a broad consensus of expert opinion in respect of drugs and their formulations and provides the physicians with carefully selected therapeutic agents of proved effectiveness which form the basis of rational drug therapy.

The National Formulary of India is an authoritative guide to prescribing, dispensing and administering medicines for healthcare professionals. It will be useful for framing national drug policies in the country. The Ministry of Health and Family Welfare, Govt. of India vide its notification F. No. X. 11035/2/06-DFQC, dated 8 th May 2008 assigned this mandatory responsibility to the Indian Pharmacopoeia Commission, Ghaziabad to publish NFI on regular basis. The IPC has published three consecutive editions of National Formulary of India since its formation.

Chronology of National Formulary of India (NFI):

The Chronology of Publication National Formulary of India is as follows:

1. The First Edition of NFI – National Formulary of India, 1960
2. The Second Edition of NFI –National Formulary of India, 1966
3. The Third Edition of NFI – National Formulary of India, 1979
4. The Fourth Edition of NFI – National Formulary of India, 2011
5. The Fifth Edition of NFI – National Formulary of India, 2016
6. The Sixth Edition of NFI (Current Edition) – National Formulary of India, 2021

Guidelines for safe Disposal of Expired Medicines[2]

Good Manufacturing Practices (GMP) and Requirements of Premises, Plant and Equipment for pharmaceutical products laid down in Schedule M of the Drugs and Cosmetics Rules, 1945 prescribe the requirements for disposal of waste including the rejected drugs. Details are as under:

1. The disposal of sewage and effluents (solid, liquid and gas) from the manufactory shall be in conformity with the requirements of Environment Pollution Control Board.
2. All bio-medical waste shall be destroyed as per the provisions of the Bio-Medical Waste (Management and Handling) Rules, 1996.
3. Additional precautions shall be taken for the storage and disposal of rejected drugs. Records shall be maintained for all disposal of waste.
4. Provisions shall be made for the proper and safe storage of waste materials awaiting disposal. Hazardous, toxic substances and flammable materials shall be stored in suitably designed and segregated, enclosed areas in conformity with Central and State Legislations.

One of the conditions of drug manufacturing license granted under the Drugs and Cosmetics Rules, 1940 is that the Licensees shall comply with the Good Manufacturing Practices (GMP) requirements prescribed in Schedule M of the said Rules. State Licensing Authorities appointed by the respective State Governments are empowered to take action in case of any violation of above requirements.

[2] https://pib.gov.in/newsite/PrintRelease.aspx?relid=178039

The Government has taken various regulatory measures to curb the misuse of antibiotics. However, no report/incidence of growing of anti-microbial resistance of drugs due to discharge of drugs and chemicals into environment has been brought to notice of this Ministry.

Conclusions

The state, as well as national governing bodies, should take strict, stringent action in managing the same, which is left behind in India which can influence the scientific method of medicine disposal. Therefore, the proper education through street play, media, conference, and awareness camps in schools and colleges regarding the disposal of drugs which is friendly with the environment can keep the universe from harmful consequence in future.

3.3 Critical Evaluation of Disposal Legislation and Consequences

It was observed that legislation is diverse among the studied countries. In a general form, laws between countries differ ranging from federal legislation to more regional regulations or even an apparent lack of regulations. Most of the country's legislations shared the establishment of collection points and the final disposal as landfills and/or incineration. The member states of the European Union stand out, since they have national regulations as well as medicine collection programs, sharing the management responsibility among all the sectors of society. Indeed, involving all social sectors in the management, such as manufacturers, distributors, prescribers, pharmacists, and public health authorities, is one way to reduce pharmaceutical pollution (Smale *et al.*, 2021).

Brazil has a recent national regulation and some regional regulations, but there is still a lack of connection between the commercial chain, *i.e.,* from the production to final disposition (Oliveira *et al.*, 2019). In addition, Brazil has many small cities not covered by the new national legislation. Moreover, awareness campaigns are crucial since ~66% of Brazilians discard expired medicines in the common garbage (Quadra *et al.*, 2019).

Among the countries with more punctual legislation, Australia and Canada have regulations at a regional scale and collection programs, but pharmaceutical disposal legislation is decentralized. Regional and local initiatives are essential, but national management may help achieve effective actions across the country. Despite being one of the pharmaceutical market leaders, Japan relies on the producers for medicine disposal management, which is risky as community participation is crucial to ensure proper disposal.

There is a concern about the most populous countries, like China and India, which seem to lack legislation. While in India, the National Formulary (NFI 2011) explains the correct disposal of drugs, an effluent from an Indian wastewater treatment contained the highest levels of pharmaceuticals reported in any effluent (Larsson *et al.*, 2007; Balakrishna *et al.*, 2017). In China, the review carried out by Liu *et al.*, (2018) showed high levels of pharmaceutical products in different environmental compartments. Most worrying is that the population is getting older, which means more drug consumption (Belloni *et al.*, 2016), and more significant pollution potential.

Although many countries have legislation, even at a regional scale, as well as çollection programs, the lack of a global standard for the collection and correct disposal of medicines has environmental impacts. aus der Beek *et al.* (2016) showed that pharmaceuticals are a global concern, although there is still a lack of data from many countries. Moreover, in general, the legislation does not include environmental monitoring and inspections to check the procedure efficiency. The pharmaceutical industry brings many benefits to humankind, but it is necessary to prevent, reduce, and manage the medicines' production, consumption, and destination. Initiatives, such as the German UBA (2018) with the "Strategic Approach to International Chemicals Management", are crucial to understand and manage pharmaceuticals globally. Organic pollutants, including some pharmaceuticals, can be transported over long distances, which can be evidenced by the detection of various compounds in non-urbanized areas, such as the poles (Gonzalez-Alonso *et al.*, 2017; Kallenborn *et al.*, 2018). Then, pharmaceuticals pollution is a global issue and needs more effort to control.

The next chapter presents study survey results and discussion on the same.

CHAPTER IV

Findings from Survey Data

4.1 Introduction

As mentioned earlier, most of the healthcare professional was not aware of proper drug disposal and their impacts. Taken together, this study was planned to introduce healthcare professionals (M.Pharm; BPharm and Nursing pursing students) and households (students of other streams like B.Ed) to assess their knowledge, practice and awareness towards safe disposal of expired drugs. This chapter presents the results of survey data.

4.2 Findings from Survey data

4.2.1 *Location of Sample Respondents*

The details on sample location as per their present stay or work are presented in Figure 4.1. It can be seen from the figures that half of the selected respondents belongs to rural areas and rest half of respondents were from urban (semi-urban and urban area) in Gujarat.

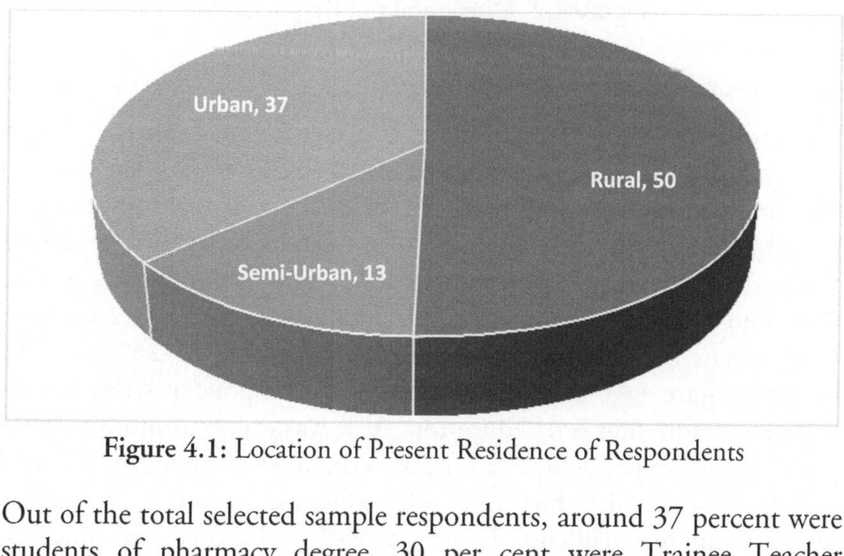

Figure 4.1: Location of Present Residence of Respondents

Out of the total selected sample respondents, around 37 percent were students of pharmacy degree, 30 per cent were Trainee Teacher students, 26 per cent were nursing diploma students and rest were others (7%) (Table 4.1 and Figure 4.2).

Table 4.1: Details of Selected Respondents Households

Sr. No.	*Respondents*	*Nos.*	*%*
1.	Pharmacy Students	143	37.1
2.	Nursing Students	100	26.0
3.	Trainee Teachers	115	29.9
4.	Others	27	7.0
		385	100

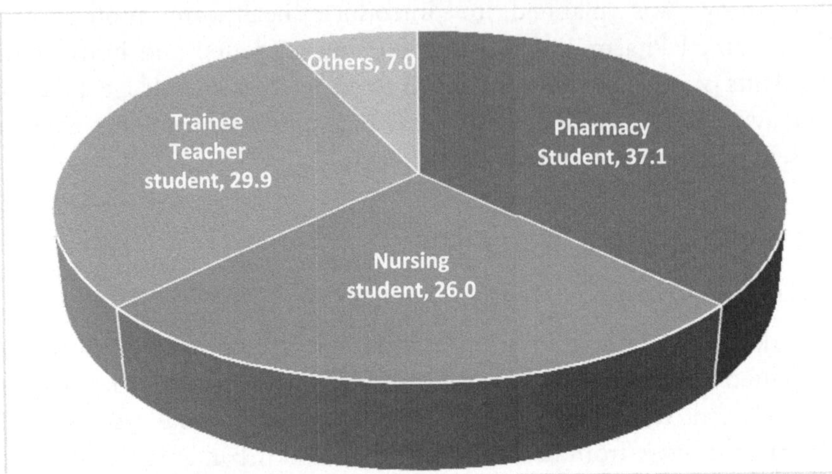

Figure 4.2: Distribution of Respondents

4.2.2 *Profile of Selected Respondents*

The profile of selected respondents is presented in Table 4.2. It can be seen from the table that dominance of female respondents (63%) was observed having more than one third share of male respondents (37%) at the overall level (Figure 4.3). Across the locality, except in semi-urban where male respondents were higher than female, picture was same as noticed at overall level. The average age of respondents was estimated to be around 21 years ranging from 21-25 across the locality (Figure 4.4). While education level of respondents was around pursuing graduation level education. As it was expected more than 98 per cent of respondents had possessed android application based mobile phone which has all facility available including immediate search about the medicine, its uses as well as disposal mechanism as prescribed by the government (Figure 4.5). It means almost everyone has available source at their tip of figures to get information related to medicine. As focus of study was to get awareness about of about use and disposal of medicines from youth and younger personals, more than 90 per cent of respondents were unmarried and rest were married one. Some of the student who are married are perusing their education for brighter future. In terms of size of family, average size of estimated to be around 5.3 person which ranges from 4.9 to 5.5 persons (Figure 4.6). One third of respondents belongs to below poverty line while rest were from above poverty line income group (Figure 4.7). The occupation of the respondents was mainly being in pursuing in education were students (Table 4.3).

Table 4.2: Profile of Selected Respondents Households

Sr. No.	*Particulars*	*Rural*	*Semi-Urban*	*Urban*	*All (%)*
1.	**Gender** (%)				
	Male	31.96	54.00	38.30	37.14
	Female	68.04	46.00	61.70	62.86
2.	Age (years)	20.81	25.28	20.60	21.31
3a.	Education (years)	13.96	14.76	13.89	14.04
3b.	Type of Mobile possess				
	Simple	2.06	2.00	0.71	1.56
	Android	97.94	98.00	99.29	98.44
4.	Marital Status				
	Single	94.33	78.00	89.36	90.39
	Married	5.67	22.00	10.64	9.61
5.	Family Size (nos)				
	Adults Male	2.45	2.02	2.27	2.33
	Adult Female	2.36	2.38	2.26	2.32
	Children	0.72	0.46	0.52	0.61
	Total	5.52	4.86	5.05	5.26
6.	Family Type (%)				
	Nuclear	20.62	40.00	36.62	29.09
	Joint	79.38	60.00	62.68	70.91

Source: Survey data.

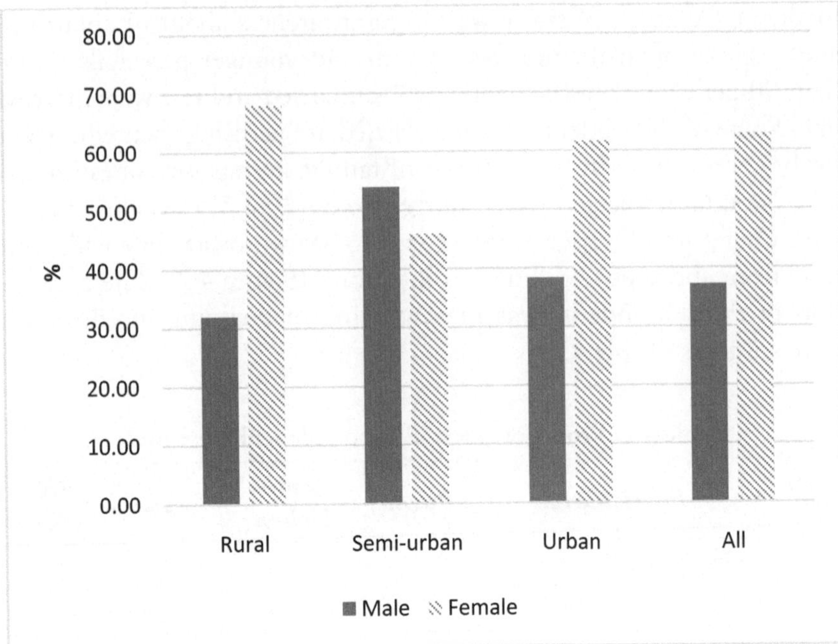

Figure 4.3: Genderwise Distribution of Selelected Respodenets

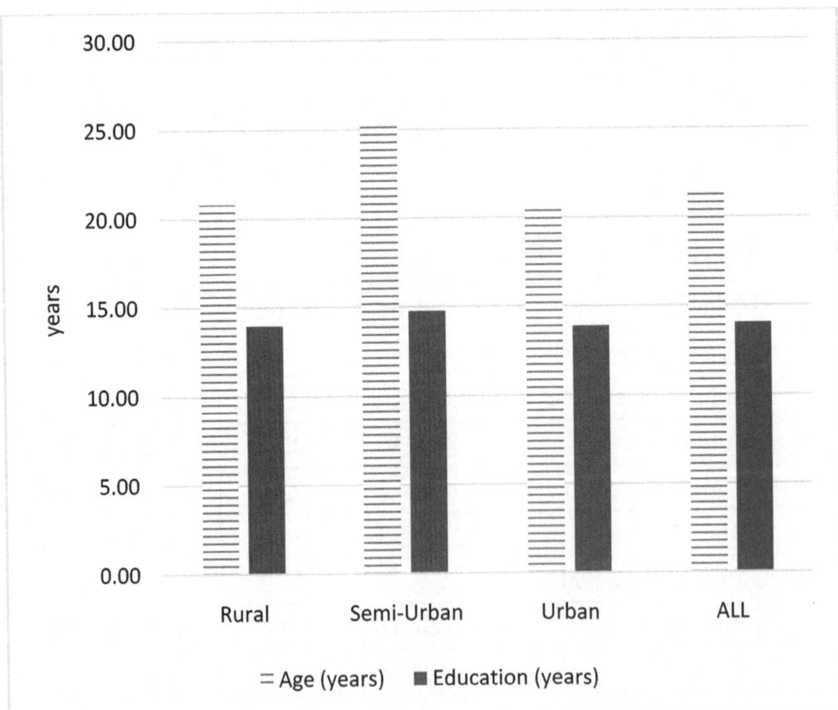

Figure 4.4: Average Age and Education of Selected Respodents (years)

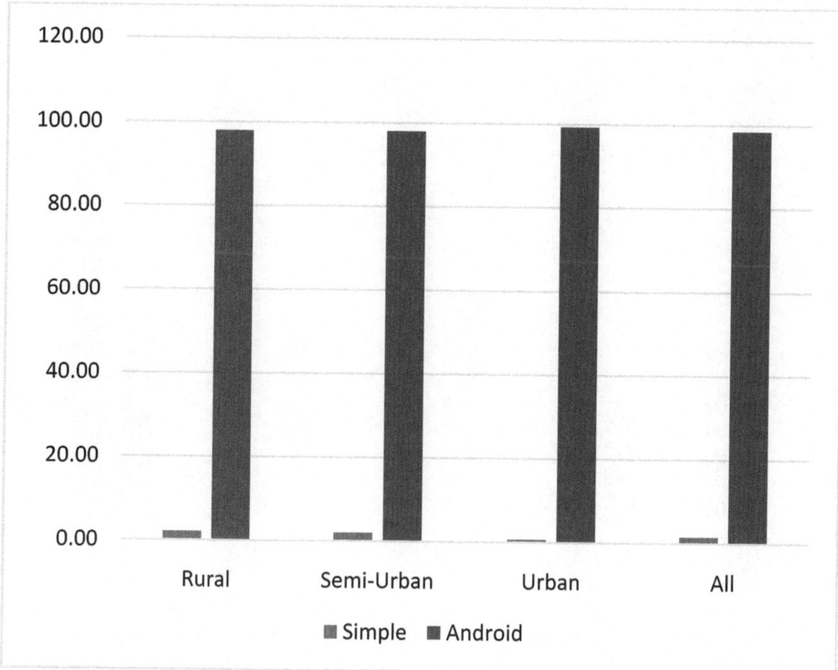

Figure 4.5: Type of Mobile Handset Possessed by the Respodents (%)

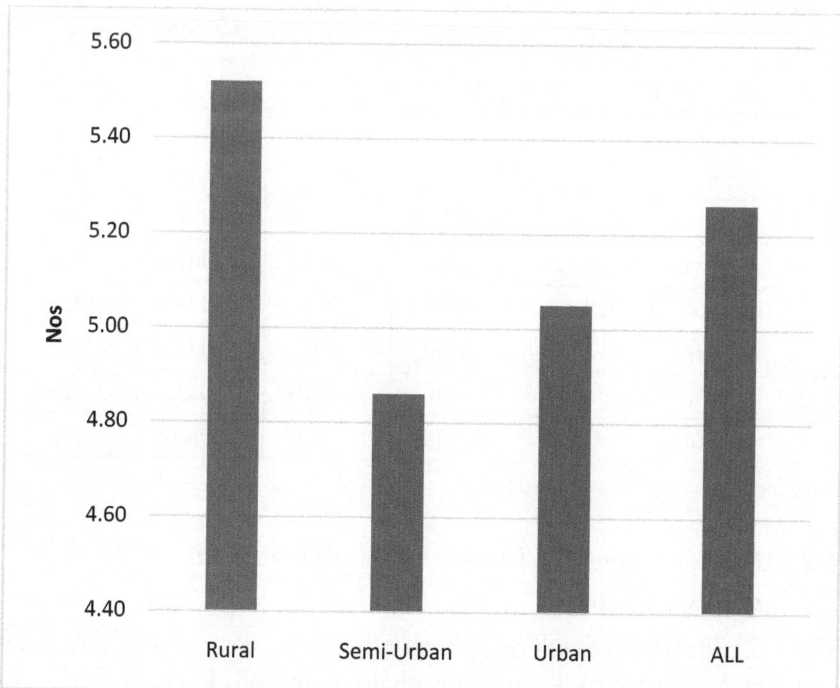

Figure 4.6: Average Family Size (Nos)

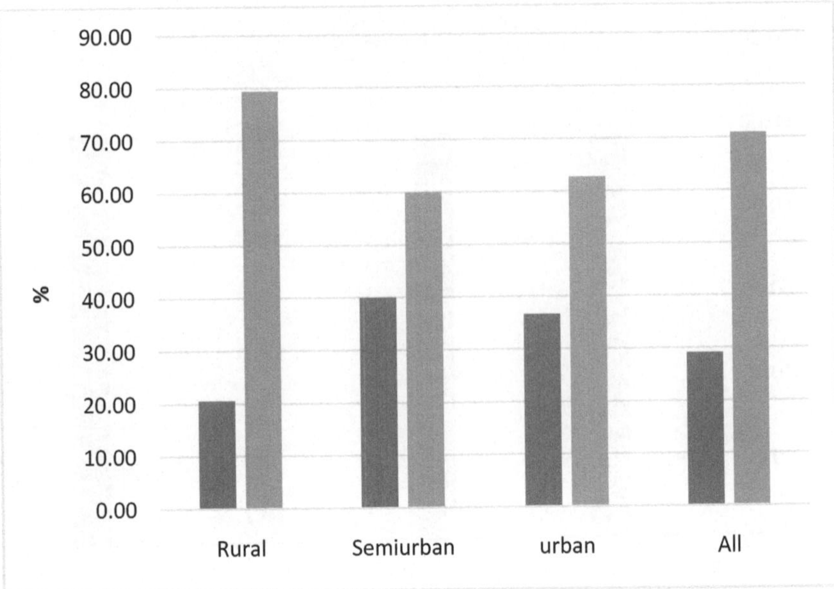

Figure 4.7: Type of Family

Table 4.3: Occupations of Selected Respondents

Sr. No.	Particulars	Rural	Semi-Urban	Urban	All (%)
1.	Student	97.94	78.00	96.45	94.81
2.	Professional	0.00	0.00	0.71	0.26
3.	Service	1.55	22.00	2.84	4.68
4.	Labour	0.00	0.00	0.00	0.00
5.	Service	0.52	0.00	0.00	0.26
6.	Crop Farming	0.00	0.00	0.00	0.00
7.	Dairy	0.00	0.00	0.00	0.00
8.	Farm labour	0.00	0.00	0.00	0.00
9.	Others	0.00	0.00	0.00	0.00

Note: Education activity as a Student.

4.2.3 *Social Category & Income Level of Households of Respondents*

The distribution of selected respondents as per social categories presented in table 4.4. indicate that at overall level, majority of respondents were from general category (39%) followed by respondents from other backward classes (29%), and Schedules tribes and Scheduled Caste (15.8% each). Across the locality, almost same kind trend was observed. In fact, rural locality has found more proper representation of SC and ST contributing more than 41 per cent share in total number of respondents (Figure 4.8). While in case of distribution of respondent's households as per their income level category, it can be seen from Table 4.5 and Figure 4.9 that tow third of total respondents were from above poverty line (66.5%) and rest were from below poverty line category (33.5%). Around 86 percent of respondents from urban and semi-urban locality were from APL category, while dominance of BPL and other category was found dominant in rural locality (53%)

Table 4.4: Social Category of Selected Respondents Households

Sr. No.	*Particulars*	*Rural*	*Semi-Urban*	*Urban*	*All (%)*
1.	Scheduled Caste	20.10	14.00	10.64	15.84
2.	Schedules Tribes	21.65	14.00	8.51	15.84
3.	OBC	26.80	32.00	31.21	29.09
4.	General/Open	31.44	40.00	49.65	39.22

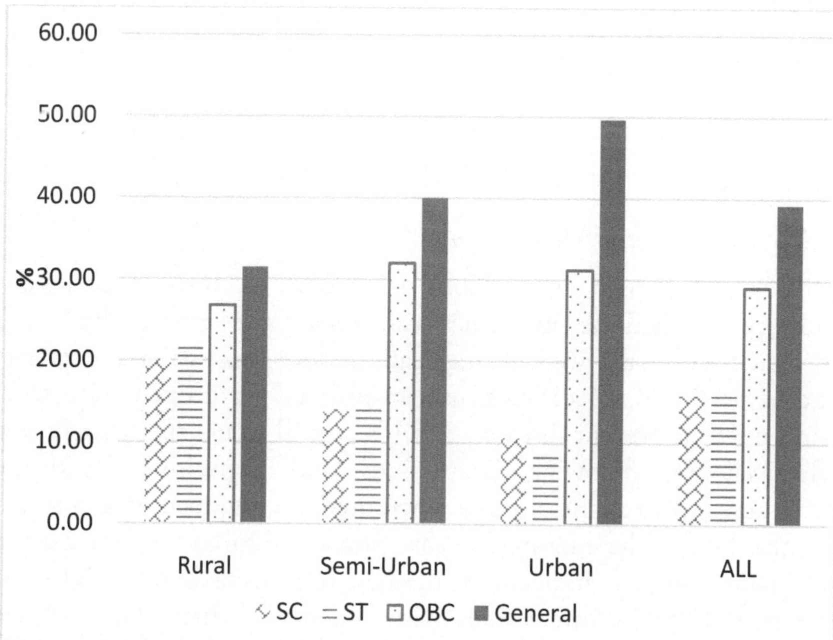

Figure 4.8: Distribution of Selected Respondents as per Social Category

Table 4.5: Income-wise Category of Selected Respondents Households

Sr. No.	*Income Category*	*Rural*	*Semi-Urban*	*Urban*	*All (%)*
1.	APL	46.91	86.00	86.52	66.49
2.	BPL & Others	53.09	14.00	13.48	33.51

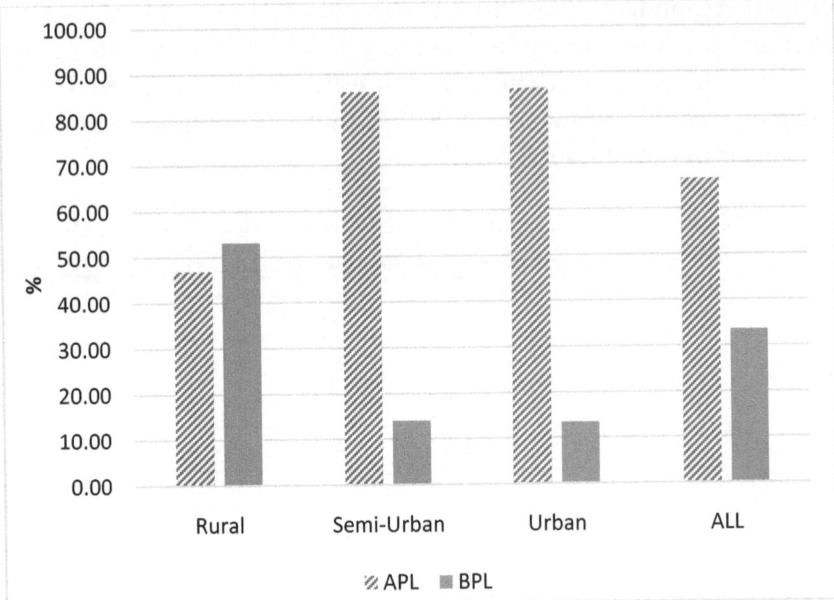

Figure 4.9: Categorisation of Respodents Households as per Income Category

4.2.4 *About Use of Medication*

Medicines are used by millions of people to treat their illness. However, sometimes medicines can cause side effects. By using medicines correctly, we can drastically reduce the risk of side effects and severe harm. Medication use involves taking drugs to diagnose, cure, treat, or prevent diseases, and it's crucial to use them safely and effectively by following instructions and consulting healthcare professionals. Medicines are safe when used as prescribed or as directed on the label. The pharmacist can provide information on how a medicine works, its indications, the best time to take it, possible side effects and/or any interactions with other medicines. The package leaflet contains important information about medicine: what it is used for, when to be extra careful, how to take it, what are the possible side effects and how to store it. It is basically necessary to read that information carefully before using the medicine. Some of the peoples go for self-medication (SM), which is a practice of using medications to treat self-diagnosed symptoms without a legitimate prescription by a health care professional.

4.2.4.1 *Frequency of Medications Storage at Household*

In order to meet the frequent need of medicine and for regular prescribed use of medicine in case of nay diseases or illness, some medicines are always kept at the home. The results on frequency of medications storage at household presented in Table 4.6 and Figure 4.10 indicate that almost half of the respondents have mentioned that they keep medicine at home (always+ often), while around 34 per cent keep medicine at home sometimes, while around 15 per cent keep it on rare case and rest were not keeping same at home.

Table 4.6: Frequency of Medications Storage at Household

Sr. No.	***Frequency***	***Rural***	***Semi-Urban***	***Urban***	***All (%)***
1.	Always	29.90	50.00	42.55	37.14
2.	Often	11.34	14.00	14.18	12.73
3.	Sometimes	39.69	24.00	29.79	34.03
4.	Rare	18.04	10.00	11.35	14.55
5.	Never	1.03	2.00	2.13	1.56

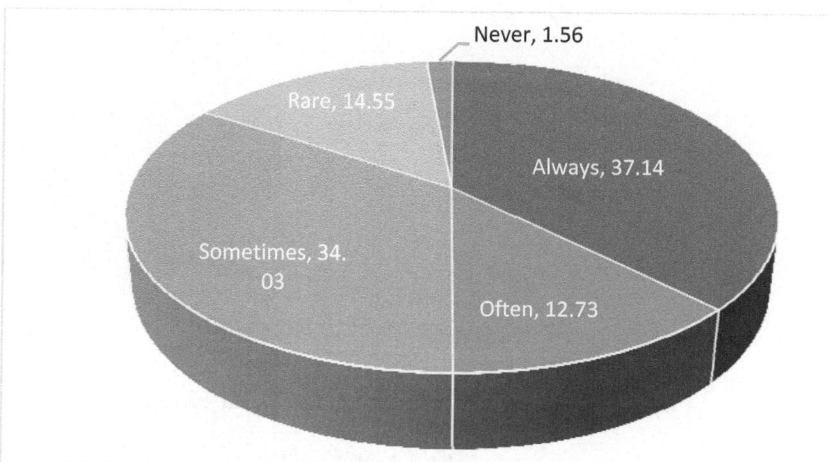

Figure 4.10: Frequency of Medicine Storage at Home

4.2.4.2 *Medicine Storage Location at Home*

Storage is crucial for the safety and quality of medicines. Medications retain their intended potency and are safer when they are store/kept at appropriate place/s. Most medications must be stored in a cool, dry place, away from direct sunlight and moisture. While few medications need refrigeration, e.g., antibiotics and insulin. Also, there is a need to keep medications out of the reach and sight of children and pets. It can be seen from Table 4.7. and Figure 4.11 that around 80 per cent of respondents have reported storing medicine in cool places such living room and bedroom, while around 13 per cent store them in refrigerators and some of them store in locker and rest of them are not clearly known about storage of medicine.

Table 4.7: Medicine Storage Location at Home

Sr. No.	*Storage Locations*	*Rural*	*Semi-Urban*	*Urban*	*All (%)*
1.	Locker	1.55	10.00	3.55	3.38
2.	Refrigerator	5.15	16.00	21.99	12.73
3.	Bedroom	34.54	24.00	29.08	31.17
4.	Living Room	53.09	46.00	42.55	48.31
5.	Don't know	5.67	4.00	2.84	4.42

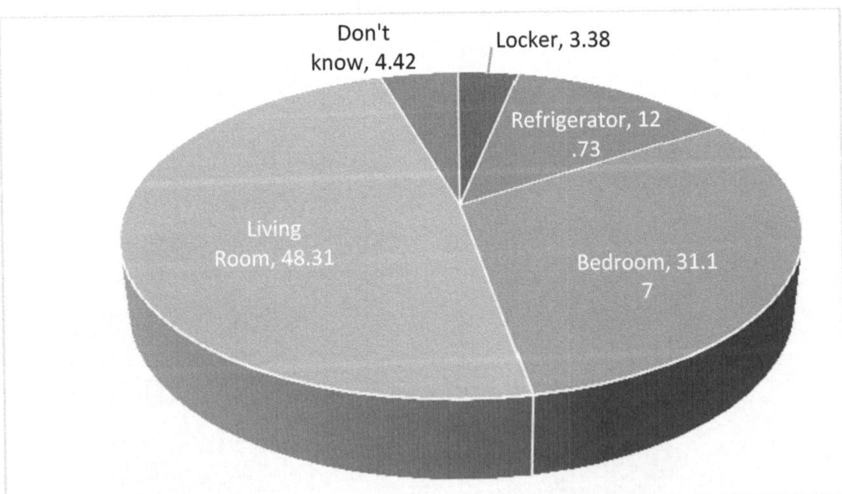

Figure 4.11: Medicine Storage Location at Home

As mentioned earlier, some of the medicines have to storage carefully at proper places. Selected respondents have mentioned that they have been storing medication away from moisture, light and high temperature as and when instructed by the pharmacist or doctor (Figure 4.12).

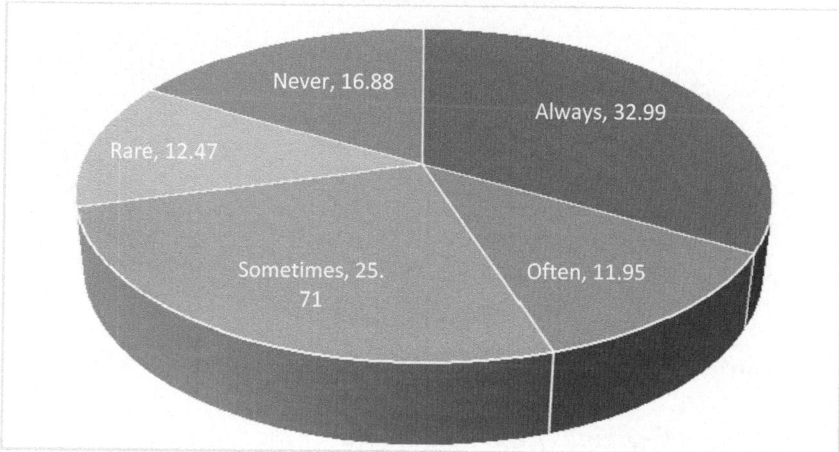

Figure 4.12: Storing of Medication away from Moisture, Light and High Temperature is Practiced in Household

4.2.4.3 *Use of Any Prescribed Medication for a Relative or a Friend*

Though it has been advocated that never give medicine to someone without their consent or try to force them to take it, sharing prescription drugs without the proper permit is absolutely illegal. It is extremely dangerous to take medicine intended for someone else's condition. Their circumstances are different, their body is different, they are probably taking another medicine too, and this medicine is chosen with that in mind. It was observed that around 12.21 per cent of respondents always share their medicines with relatives or friends, while 6.23 per cent respondents do it often and 38 per cent of respondents do it sometimes.

Table 4.8: Use of Any Prescribed Medication for a Relative or a Friend

Sr. No.	***Frequency***	***Responses (%)***
1.	Always	12.21
2.	Often	6.23
3.	Sometimes	38.44
4.	Rare	22.34
5.	Never	20.78

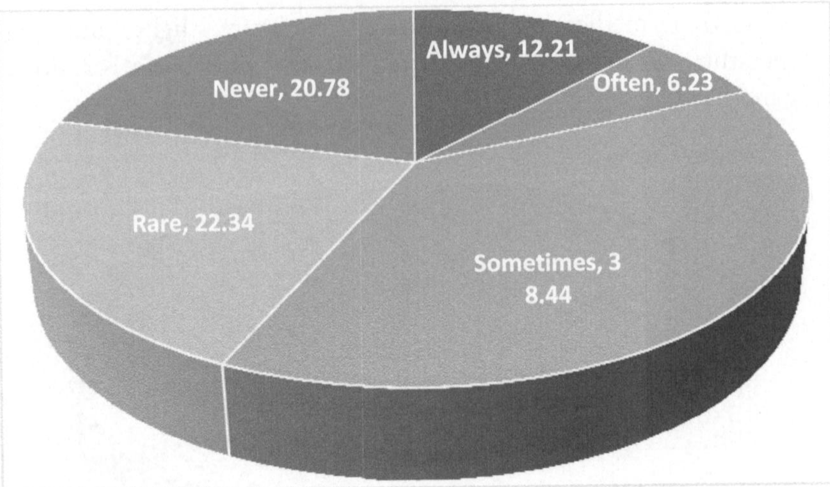

Figure 4.13: Use of Prescribed Medication for a Relative or a Friend

4.2.4.4 *Act of Checking of Expiration Date of the Medicine before Buying it*

Checking the expiration date of medicine before purchasing is crucial for ensuring its safety and effectiveness, as using expired medication can be harmful or ineffective. It can be seen from Table 4.9 and Figure 4.14 that around 87 per cent of selected respondents have reported that they check expiry date printed on medicine while purchasing it which is welcome to note. It has been also advocated that before administering any medication, it should always verify the expiry date to ensure patient safety and efficacy. Expired medications can become ineffective or even harmful due to degradation or bacterial growth. It can be seen from Table 4.10 and Figure 4.15 that around 81 percent of respondents have reported that they verify the expiry date on medicine before administering medication.

Table 4.9: Frequency of Checking of Expiration Date of the Medicine before Buying it

Sr. No.	*Frequency*	*Rural*	*Semi-Urban*	*Urban*	*All (%)*
1.	Always	86.60	86.00	86.52	86.49
2.	Often	2.58	8.00	2.84	3.38
3.	Sometimes	3.09	2.00	4.96	3.64
4.	Rare	4.12	2.00	4.26	3.90
5.	Never	3.61	2.00	1.42	2.60

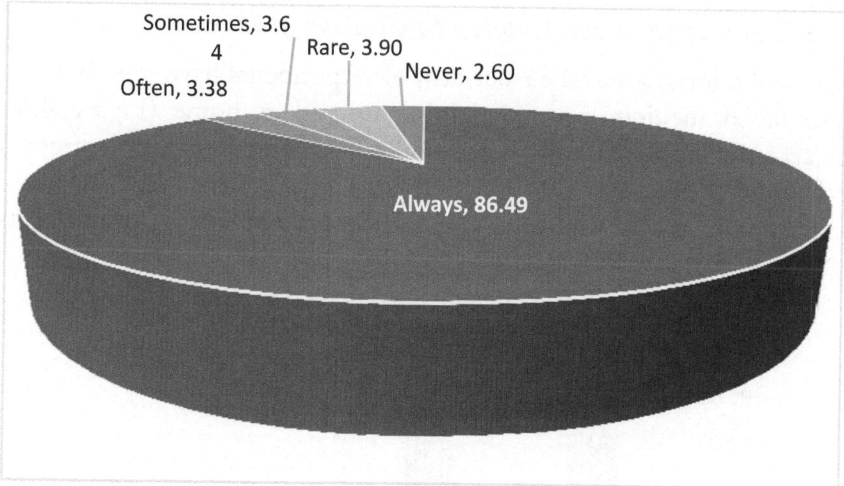

Figure 4.14: Act of Checking the Expiration Date of the Medicine before Buying it (%)

Table 4.10: Verification of Expiry Date before Administering Medications

Sr. No.	*Frequency*	*Rural*	*Semi-Urban*	*Urban*	*All (%)*
1.	Always	79.90	86.00	80.14	80.78
2.	Often	6.19	4.00	2.13	4.42
3.	Sometimes	3.61	4.00	2.84	3.38
4.	Rare	8.76	6.00	12.06	9.61
5.	Never	1.55	2.00	2.84	2.08

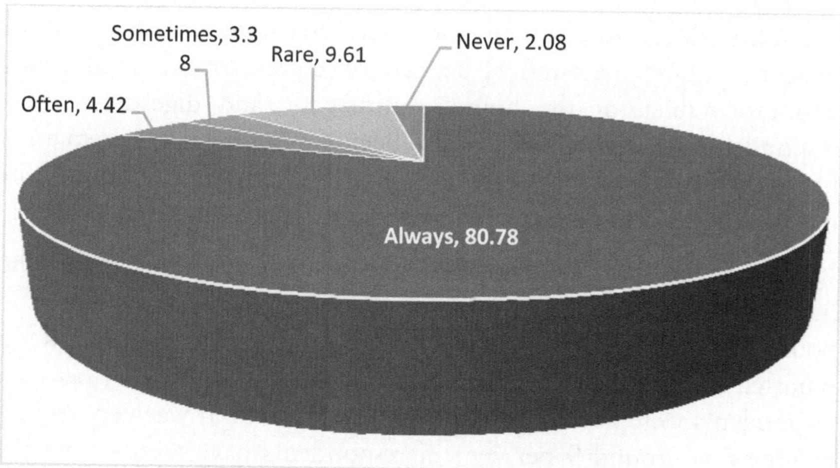

Figure 4.15: Verification of Expiry Date before Administering Medications (%)

4.2.5 *About Used and Expired Medication at Home*

At overall level, around 88 per cent of respondents have reported that purchased medicines are remaining unused at home (Figure 4.6). Across the locality, the highest number of respondents were observed in Semi-urban area (90%) followed by around 89 per cent respondents from rural area and the lowest number of respondents (86%) reported having medicine at the home.

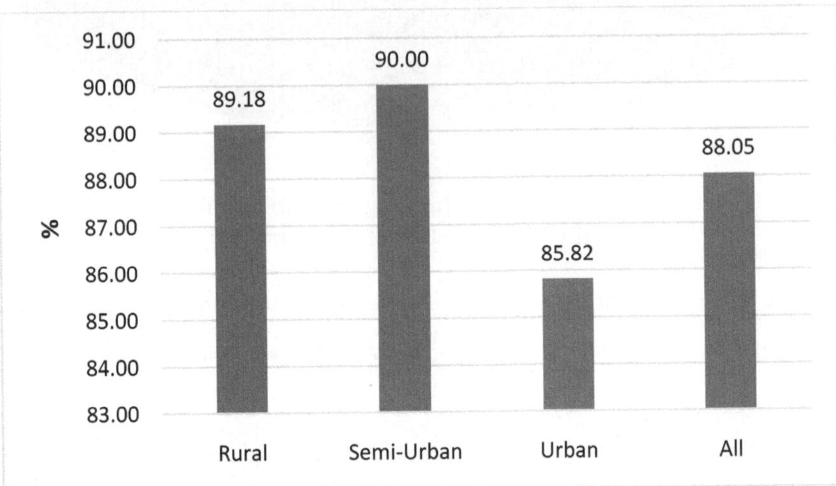

Figure 4.16: Purchased Medicines Remaining Unused at Home among Household

It can be seen from table 4.11 that 68 per cent of respondents had painkiller tablets (Analgesic medicine) at their home as usual required medicine at home. Around 41 per cent of respondents reported having antibiotic tablets at the home. Antidiabetic and digestions (41% respondents) related tablets are also been among medicines remain at home. While few of them (18–19%) also had, power and liquid state medicine related to digestion was also been reported unused at home.

It can be seen from Figure 4.17 that out of respondents those who have reported, the average number of unused medications stored in household are presented in around 66 per cent of respondents reported having 0 to 5 medicines at home while around 18 per cent respondents were having 6–10 medicines at home. It was very strange to note that around 9 per cent of respondents have reported having more than 20 medicine at home. Around 88 per cent of respondents have reported having prescribed medicine at the home while 42 percent of residents non-prescribed medicines at home. Thus, medicines have been kept at home of both the nature (prescribed and non-prescribed).

Table 4.11: Details on Type of Medication Remaining Unused at Home among Household

Sr, No.	*Types of Medicines*	*Tablets*	*Capsule*	*Powder*	*Liquid/ Syrup*	*Other*
1.	Analgesic (pain killer)	68.05	12.99	2.86	11.69	9.09
2.	Antibiotic (destroying bacteria and curing infections)	41.04	11.17	5.45	11.95	6.75
3.	Antihypertensive (for hypertension)	29.35	10.13	4.68	4.94	5.97
4.	Antidiabetic (blood glucose control)	40.78	8.83	9.35	10.39	8.31
5.	Digestion (for digest and constipation)	40.52	13.51	18.18	18.96	10.13
6.	Skin disease (dermatology)	35.06	7.79	9.09	11.95	21.04
7.	Other medication	36.88	4.42	3.38	3.90	15.06

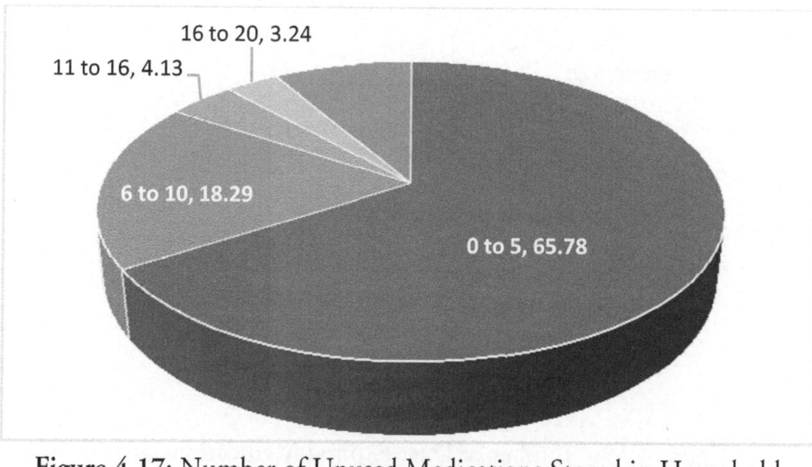

Figure 4.17: Number of Unused Medications Stored in Household

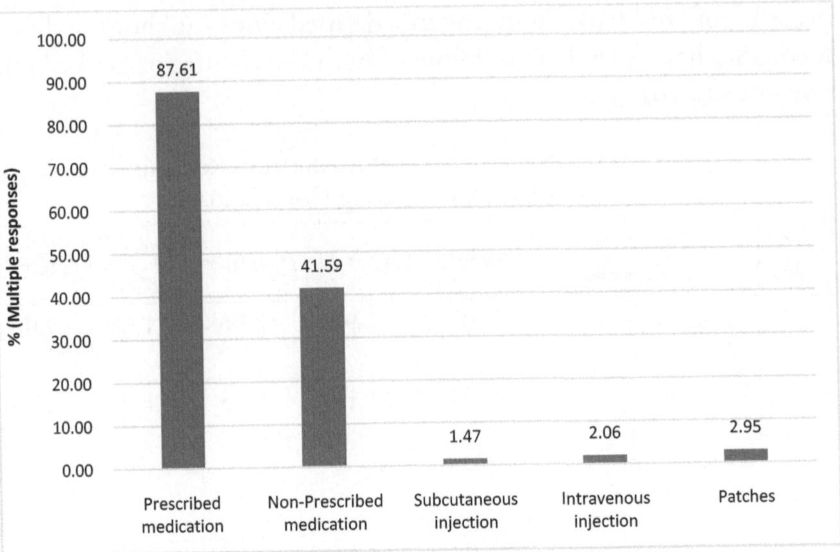

Figure 4.18: Classes of Unused Medications that are in Your Household (%, multiple responses)

In case of date expired medicines, as per responses received, around 89 per cent respondents have mentioned of having 0–5 date expired medicines, while hardly one per cent have reported having more than 20 date expired medicines (Figure 4.19). The medicines which was date expired was mostly prescribed one (60%) followed by 29 per cent of non-prescribed medicines (Figure 4.20).

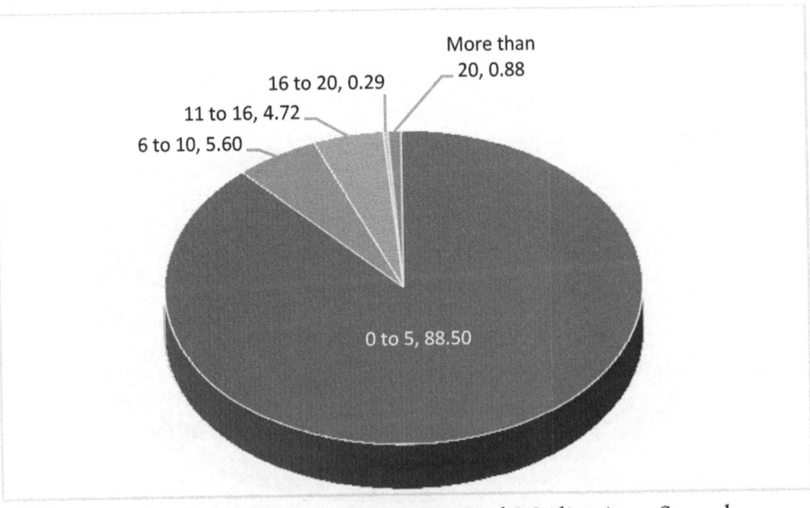

Figure 4.19: Number of Date Expired Medications Stored in Household (%, responded)

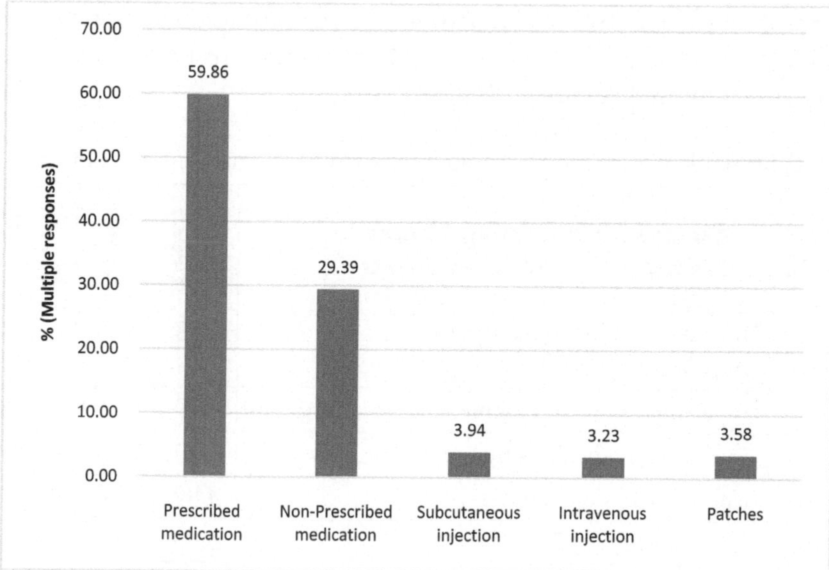

Figure 4.20: Classes of Date Expired Medications that are in Your Household (%, multiple responses)

4.2.6 *Reasons for Keeping Purchased Medicine Unused at Home*

Medicine use can be influenced by several factors. Factors influencing the use of medicines in the community include knowledge about use, the cost of medicines, regulatory systems, cultural factors, community beliefs and communication with prescribers among others. These factors play out at different levels including houschold and community. The way medicines are used is also influenced by individual beliefs about them, which may have been shaped by members of the immediate family and those in extended family networks at household level. The community is the immediate context in which individuals and families deal with their health problems. People talk to each other about therapies, creating and reinforcing existing medicine use cultures, and they rely on local sources of medicines. In order to address the problem of irrational use of medicines, health planners and administrators require specific information on the types, extent and the reasons of irrational use of medicines. The major reason cited by the respondents for keeping purchased medicine unused at home was disease or condition got resolved or patient recovered (69%) followed by change of medication by the doctor (49%) and forgetting to take medicine (40%). While some of them have reported medicine due to experiencing side effect

(33%) and bitter taste (36%). Around 31 per cent respondent reported that due to change of doctor or starting of another treatment, medicine remained unused (Figure 4.21, Table 4.12).

Table 4.12: Reasons for Keeping Purchased Medicine Unused at Home

Sr, No.	*Reasons for Possessing Unused Medication (multiple responses)*	*Rural*	*Semi-Urban*	*Urban*	*Grand Total*
1.	Disease or condition resolve/ symptoms improved	35.06	8.83	24.68	68.57
2.	Forgetting to take medicine	22.60	5.19	11.69	39.48
3.	Change of medication by the doctor	24.94	6.23	17.92	49.09
4.	Experiencing side-effect	17.92	3.90	10.65	32.47
5.	Taste is bitter	21.30	3.90	10.65	35.84
6.	Busy schedule	13.25	3.12	9.61	25.97
7.	Change of doctor/Change to another treatment	16.62	2.34	11.69	30.65
8.	Excess quantity supplied	12.21	2.86	6.75	21.82
9.	Inconvenience/Difficulty following instructions	4.94	0.26	1.82	7.01
10.	Medicine label had unclear instruction	7.79	2.08	3.90	13.77

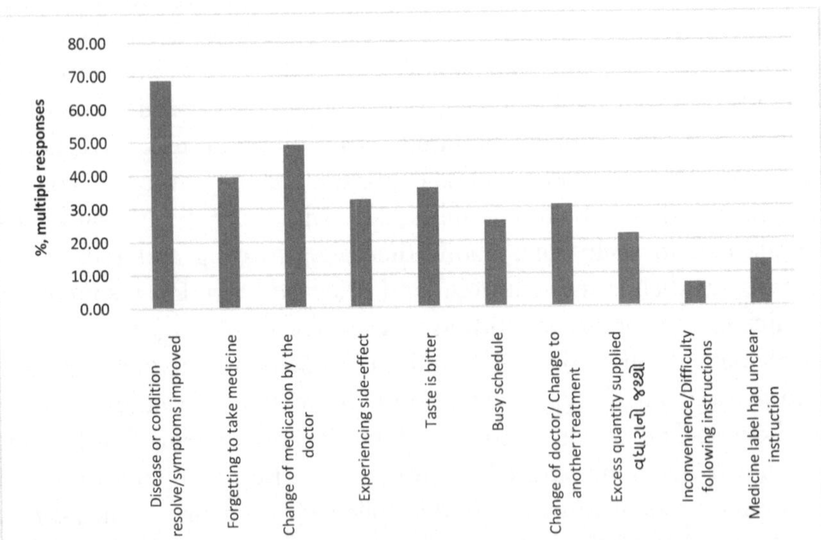

Figure 4.21: Reasons for Possessing Unused Medication

4.2.7 *Knowledge on Disposal of Unused and Expired Medication*

As we have discussed in earlier chapters, majority of the consumers remain unaware about the disposal of unused or expired medicines. Improper disposal of expired and unused medications has several consequences such as environmental pollution, childhood poisoning, negative impact on wildlife, and development of drug-resistant micro-organisms. The details on knowledge on disposal of unused and expired medication of selected respondents are presented in Table 4.13 and Figure 4.22. It can be seen that around 64 per cent of respondents agreed that they are aware about the fact that misused/repeated change or not complete antibiotics may cause drug resistance. While 37 per cent respondents knew about "drug-take-back system. Around 67 percent of respondents separate unused medicine before disposal. While, in case of date expired medicines, 23–24 per cent respondents know about medication waste and they read medicines disposal instruction and they have you ever followed medicines disposal instruction. These respondents must have from the pharmaceutical and nursery diploma holders background who have received some information about the disposal of same. Around 67 per cent of respondents knew that improper disposal of unused and expired medicines can affect the environment and health. Only one third of them have reported receiving education regarding safe disposal of medication. Very few of them reported seeking information from official resources safe disposals of medications.

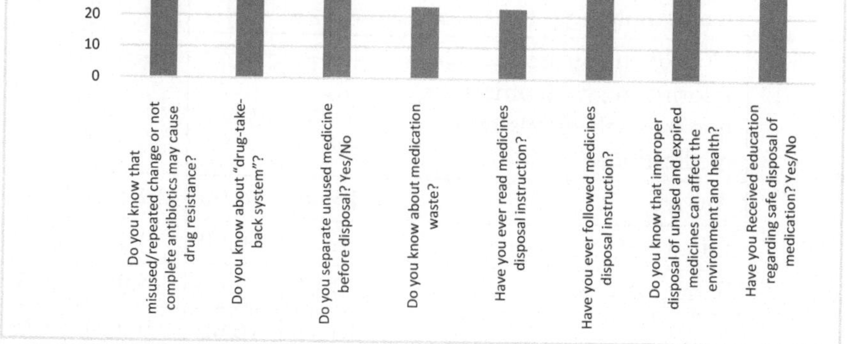

Figure 4.22: Knowledge on Disposal of Unused and Expired Medication (%)

Table 4.13: Details on Knowledge on Disposal of Unused and Expired Medication

Sr, No.	***Reasons for Possessing Unused Medication (% Yes responses)***	***Rural***	***Semi-Urban***	***Urban***	***Grand Total***
A.	**Unused**				
1.	Do you know that misused/ repeated change or not complete antibiotics may cause drug resistance?	61.3	78.0	62.4	63.9
2.	Do you know about "drug-take-back system"?	39.7	22.0	38.3	36.9
3.	Do you separate unused medicine before disposal? Yes/No	66.5	74.0	63.8	66.5
B.	**Date Expired**				
1.	Do you know about medication waste?	21.65	12.00	28.37	22.86
2.	Have you ever read medicines disposal instruction?	23.71	18.00	21.99	22.34
3.	Have you ever followed medicines disposal instruction?	36.08	36.00	44.68	39.22
4.	Do you know that improper disposal of unused and expired medicines can affect the environment and health?	70.10	64.00	64.54	67.27
5.	Have you Received education regarding safe disposal of medication? Yes/No	28.87	32.00	41.13	33.77
6.	How often you seek information from official resources safe disposals of medications				
	Always	15.46	6.00	19.15	15.58
	Often	6.70	10.00	9.93	8.31
	Sometimes	30.41	16.00	14.89	22.86
	Rare	10.31	16.00	9.93	10.91
	Never	37.11	52.00	46.10	42.34

4.2.8 *Disposal Practice of Unused Medicines among Households*

Among the selected respondents' household, common disposal practices for unused and expired medicines include throwing them in the garbage/trash as reported by 74 per cent of respondents, while 27 per cent of respondents have disposed it by burning followed 22 per cent of respondents have flushed them down the toilet or sink. It indicates significant portion also unaware of proper disposal methods (table 4.14 and Figure 4.23).

Table 4.14: Details on Disposal Practice of Unused Medicines among Households

Sr, No.	*Suggested Actions (% Yes responses)*	*Rural*	*Semi-Urban*	*Urban*	*Grand Total*
1.	Throwing them away in household garbage	74.74	68.00	75.18	74.03
2.	Donating them to hospital	0.00	0.00	0.00	0.00
3.	Giving them to friends or relatives	33.51	30.00	29.79	31.69
4.	Returning them back to pharmacy	19.07	34.00	26.24	23.64
5.	Returning to Hospital	22.16	16.00	21.28	21.04
6.	Keeping them at home until expired	35.05	30.00	29.08	32.21
7.	Flushing them in toilet	27.32	18.00	15.60	21.82
8.	Burning them	30.41	22.00	22.70	26.49
9.	Lowering the number of prescribed medicines by doctors	27.32	24.00	22.70	25.19
10.	Give/ donate medication to other people	0.00	0.00	0.00	0.00
11.	I do not dispose medication	0.52	0.00	0.00	0.26

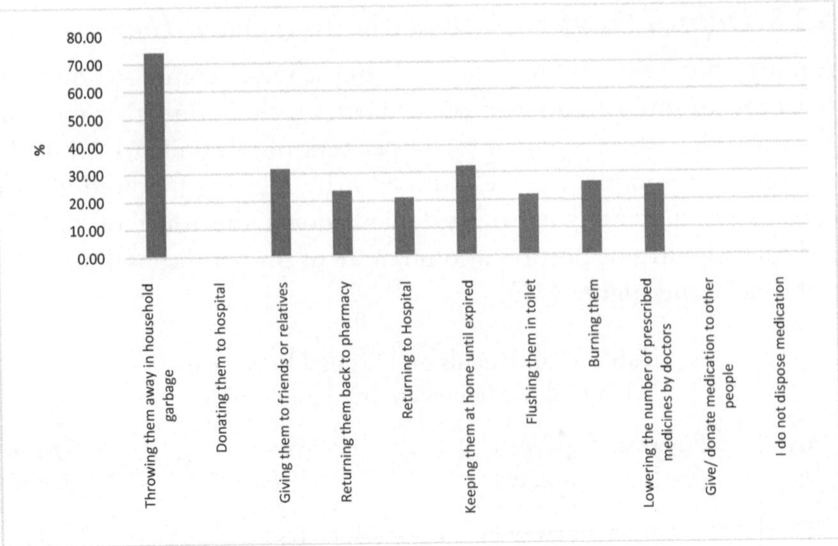

Figure 4.23: Disposal Practice of Unused Medicines among Households

In case of date-expired medicine disposal practises, around 76 per cent of respondents reported throwing them away in household garbage followed by 22 per cent respondents flushing them in toilets. Around 27 per cent respondent mentioned that date-expired medicines were disposed by burning the (table 4.15 and Figure 4.24).

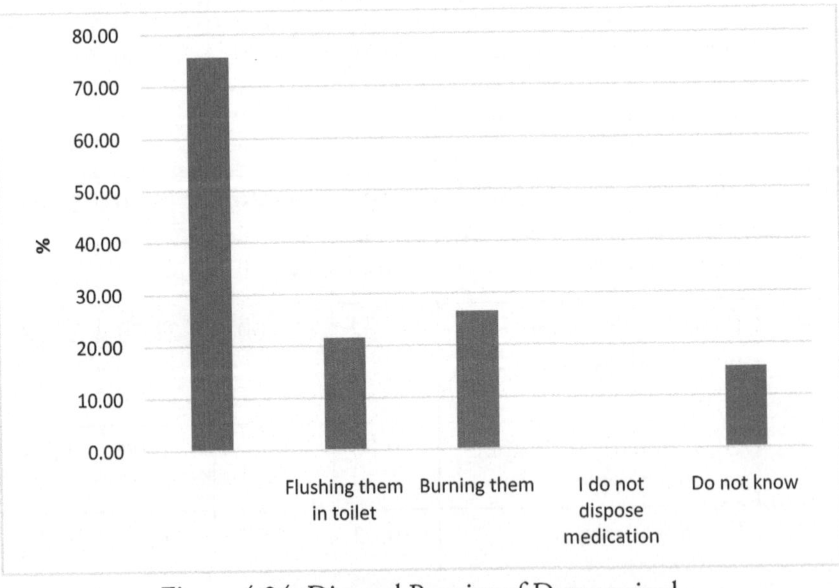

Figure 4.24: Disposal Practice of Date-expired Medicines among Households

Table 4.15: Details on Disposal Practice of Date-expired Medicines among Households

Sr, No.	*Responses as Yes (% to respective locality)*	*Rural*	*Semi-Urban*	*Urban*	*Grand Total*
1.	Throwing them away in household garbage	73.20	74.00	79.43	75.58
2.	Flushing them in toilet	22.16	22.00	20.57	21.56
3.	Burning them	32.47	20.00	20.57	26.49
4.	I do not dispose medication	0.00	0.00	0.00	0.00
5.	Do not know	16.49	12.00	15.60	15.58

4.2.9 *Perceptions Towards Disposal of Unused/Expired Medicines*

The respondent's perceptions about disposal of unused and date-expired medicines in presented in Table 4.16. It can be seen from table that all the respondents agreed opined that unused medicines should not be thrown into dustbins and burning of expired medicines can release toxic substances which can be inhaled by the people. Also, all agreed for the fact that there should be a public awareness program

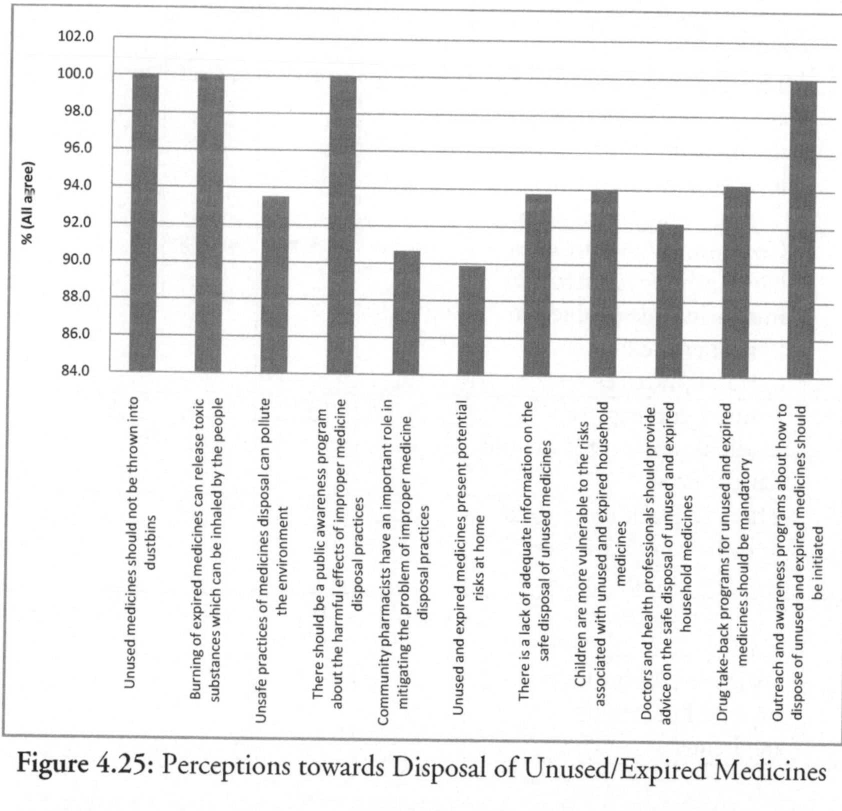

Figure 4.25: Perceptions towards Disposal of Unused/Expired Medicines

about the harmful effects of improper medicine disposal practices. Around 97 percent of respondents opined that unsafe practices of medicines disposal can pollute the environment. Around 93 per cent of respondents agreed on the fact that community pharmacists have an important role in mitigating the problem of improper medicine disposal practices (Figure 4.25).

Table 4.16: Perceptions towards Disposal of Unused/Expired Medicines (%)

Sr, No.	*Statement*	*Strengly Agree*	*Slightly Agree*	*Agree*	*Disagree*	*Strongly Disgaree*
1.	Unused medicines should not be thrown into dustbins	51.69	10.13	38.18	0.00	0.00
2.	Burning of expired medicines can release toxic substances which can be inhaled by the people	35.84	13.25	50.91	0.00	0.00
3.	Unsafe practices of medicines disposal can pollute the environment	42.86	10.91	39.74	2.86	3.64
4.	There should be a public awareness program about the harmful effects of improper medicine disposal practices	43.12	11.95	44.94	0.00	0.00
5.	Community pharmacists have an important role in mitigating the problem of improper medicine disposal practices	36.36	13.51	40.78	6.49	2.86
6.	Unused and expired medicines present potential risks at home	28.57	13.25	48.05	7.53	2.60
7.	There is a lack of adequate information on the safe disposal of unused medicines	33.25	9.09	51.43	6.23	0.00
8.	Children are more vulnerable to the risks associated with unused and expired household medicines	40.00	10.91	43.12	3.90	2.08

Sr, No.	Statement	Strengly Agree	Slightly Agree	Agree	Disagree	Strongly Disgaree
9.	Doctors and health professionals should provide advice on the safe disposal of unused and expired household medicines	40.00	13.51	38.70	5.45	2.34
10.	Drug take-back programs for unused and expired medicines should be mandatory	30.91	41.82	21.56	5.71	0.00
11.	Outreach and awareness programs about how to dispose of unused and expired medicines should be initiated	36.36	9.61	54.03	0.00	0.00

4.2.10 *Actions to Minimize or Control the Hazardous Effect of Unused and Expired Medicines*

Safely dispose of unused or expired medicines before they can do harm. There are many ways to get rid of them. The 72 per cent of respondents suggested to providing proper guidance to the consumer, while 63 per cent opined that same can be done consuming the same as per doctor advice (Table 4.17 and Figure 4.26). Around 60 per cent

Table 4.17: Details on Suggested Actions to Minimize or Control the Hazardous Effect of Unused and Expired Medicines

Sr, No.	Suggestions (% Yes)	Rural	Semi-Urban	Urban	Grand Total
1.	By providing proper guidance to the consumer	69.07	82.00	72.34	71.95
2.	By prescribing in quantities and for duration that ensure patient compliance	57.22	58.00	63.12	59.48
3.	By donating the unused medicines	32.99	54.00	41.13	38.70

Sr, No.	*Suggestions (% Yes)*	*Rural*	*Semi-Urban*	*Urban*	*Grand Total*
4.	By depositing unused medicine in nearby Public Health Centre	57.73	52.00	52.48	55.06
5.	By consuming the same as per doctor advice	67.01	56.00	59.57	62.86
6.	Lowering the number of prescribed medicines by doctor	41.75	38.00	41.13	41.04

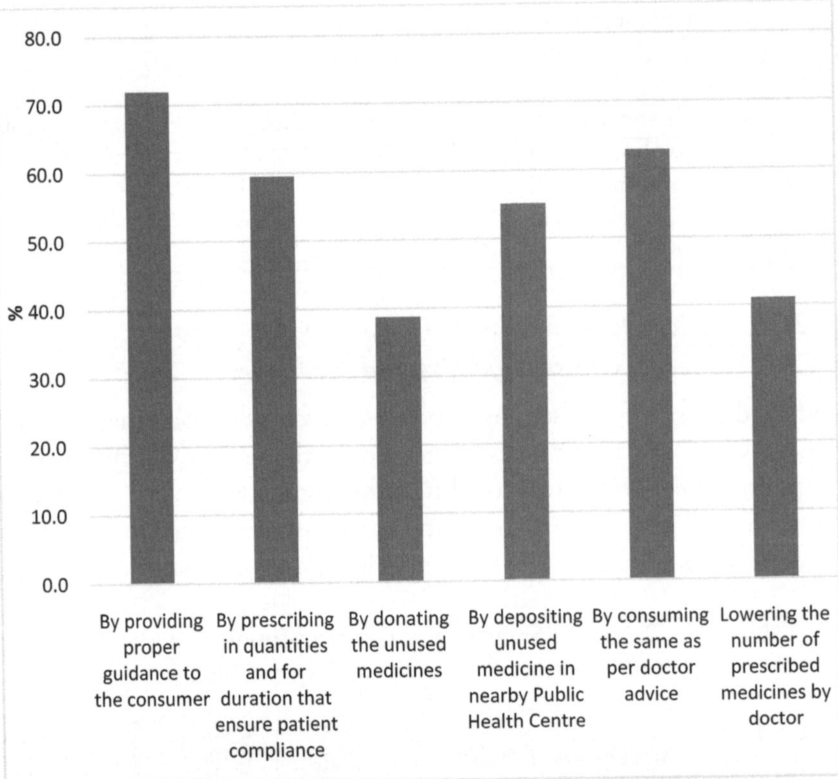

Figure 4.26: Actions to Minimize or Control the Hazardous Effect of Unused and Expired Medicines (%)

of respondents suggested to prescribe in quantities and for duration that ensure patient compliance while 55 per cent suggested to deposit unused medicine in nearby Public Health Centre. Around 39-41 per cent of respondents have suggested to donate the unused medicines and also by lowering the number of prescribed medicines by doctor.

4.2.11 *Bodies Responsible for Creation of Awareness about Disposal of Unused and Expired Medication*

The respondents were asked to mentioned about their perception about bodies responsible for creation of awareness about disposal of unused and expired medication (Tale 4.18 & Figure 4.27). The 61 per cent respondent opined that government mechanism (health department and related sections) followed by health bureau (57%) should create awareness about proper disposal of unused and expired medications. Around 55 per cent respondents noted that awareness need to be spearheaded by pharmacists followed by healthcare professionals, i.e. physician and doctors (50%).

Table 4.18: Bodies Responsible for Creation of Awareness about Disposal of Unused and Expired Medication

Sr, No.	***Responses (% Yes)***	***Rural***	***Semi-Urban***	***Urban***	***Grand Total***
1.	Physician/Doctor	50.52	56.00	47.52	50.13
2.	Pharmacist/Chemist shop	51.03	60.00	57.45	54.55
3.	Pharmaceutical industries	31.44	42.00	36.17	34.55
4.	Every health professional	42.78	42.00	41.84	42.34
5.	Government /government mechanism	57.73	54.00	66.67	60.52
6.	NGOs	30.41	38.00	38.30	34.29
7.	Health bureau	59.79	46.00	56.74	56.88
8.	Environment agency	37.11	44.00	38.30	38.44
9.	Drug regulatory agency	36.60	48.00	38.30	38.70

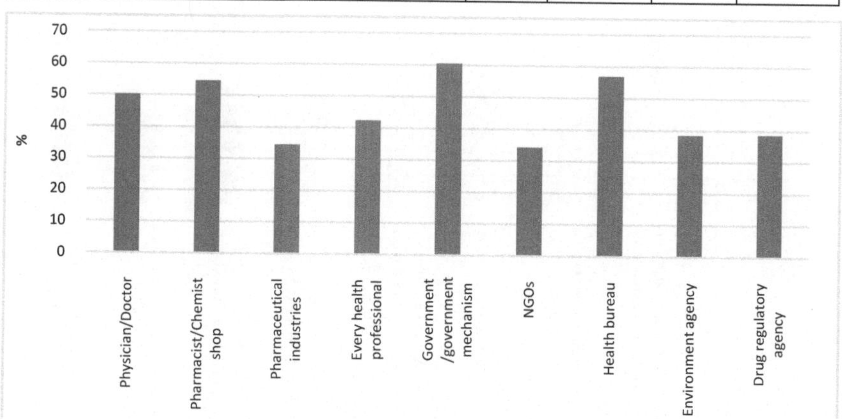

Figure 4.27: Bodies Responsible for Creation of Awareness about Disposal of Unused and Expired Medication

The respondents were asked to suggest best/preferred method for creation of awareness about disposal of unused and expired medication. Around 87 per cent of respondents have suggested to arrange awareness program in every village/hospital, while around 65–67 percent of respondents opined to create awareness through print (newspaper/ magazines), air and electronic media (Program on TV, Radio) and digital (Youtube, Facebook, Whatsup, instagram) media. While 61 per cent of respondents suggested to include topic on use and disposal pf medicine in school curriculum

Table 4.19: Best/Preferred method for Creation of Awareness about Disposal of Unused and Expired Medication

Sr, No.	*Responses (% Yes)*	*Rural*	*Semi-Urban*	*Urban*	*Grand Total*
1.	Awareness program in every village/hospital	88.66	72.00	90.07	87.01
2.	Hoardings/Posters/Pamplets	41.24	52.00	44.68	43.90
3.	Newspaper/Magazines	67.01	62.00	67.38	66.49
4.	Air and Electronic media (Program on TV, Radio)	67.01	60.00	63.83	64.94
5.	Digital Media (Youtube, Facebook, Whatsup, instagram)	65.98	74.00	63.12	65.97
6.	Introducing the topic on School Curriculum	61.86	56.00	61.70	61.04
7.	Mobile dialer tone like Covid19	45.88	44.00	39.72	43.38
8.	Text messages on Mobile	51.03	44.00	43.97	47.53

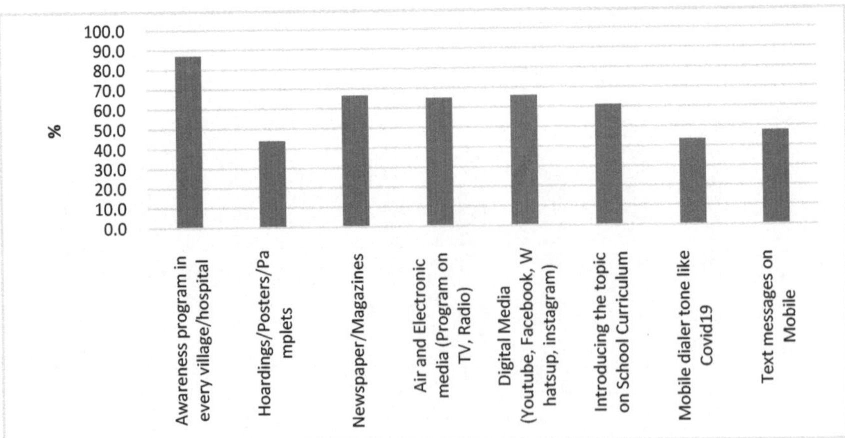

Figure 4.28: Best/Preferred Method for Creation of Awareness about Disposal of Unused and Expired Medication

4.2.12 *Suggestions*

All the selected respondents perceived that there is a need for a program to collect unused medicines from home. All the selected respondents also agreed that consumers should be made more aware about donation of medicines and hazards of unsafe disposal & methods of safe disposal (table 4.20)

Table 4.20: Perceptions about Collection Point and Awareness Programs

Sr. No.	*Perception*	*Yes (%)*
1.	Do you think that there is a need for a program to collect unused medicines from home?	100
2.	Do you think that consumers should be made more aware about donation of medicines	100
3.	Do you think that consumers should be made more aware about hazards of unsafe disposal & methods of safe disposal?	100

Around 55 percent of respondents have suggested to keep medicine at proper places followed by 35 percent respondents suggested to return unused medicine to chemist followed by 29 per cent respondents suggested to organise awareness programs at schools to improve awareness of consumers regarding safe disposal of medicines.

Table 4.21: Suggestions Made by the Respondents

Sr. No.	*Suggestions*	*Yes (%)*
1.	Keep medicine at proper place	55.06
2.	Return to chemist	34.81
3.	Awareness @ school	29.09
4.	Collection point	1.82
5.	Donate to needy people	0.52
6.	Awareness through U tube & social media	0.78
7.	Awareness programs	2.60

4.3 Response of Pharmacists

Pharmacists are key players in the pharmaceutical supply chain and are in a position to contribute to the reduction of medication waste and for creating awareness about proper disposal of medicines by educating patients, participating in take-back programs, and implementing effective inventory management practices within pharmacies. The survey results indicate that majority of the pharmacist were from Urban area (53%) followed by semi urban (40%) and rest were from rural areas (table 4.22). All the pharmacists were registered drug shoppers. Around three fifth of pharmacists possess diploma level of education while rest of two fifth were graduated in pharmacy/science subject. Out of total selected pharmacist, 73 per cent were male and rest were female respondents (27%). The average age of respondent pharmacist were estimated to be 34 years and having experience of around 11 years in pharmacy.

Table 4.22: Profile of Selected Pharmacists

Sr. No.	*Parameters*	*Responses*
1.	Locality (%)	
	Village	6.70
	Semi Urban	40.00
	Urban	53.30
2.	About Registration (%)	
	Registered Pharmacists	100.0
	Unregistered Pharmacists	0.00
3.	Education level	
	D. Pham	60.00
	B.Pharm/Bachelor	40.00
4.	Gender (male/Female) (%)	
	Male	73.33
	Female	26.67
5.	Age (years)	34.2
6.	Experience of Pharmacy (years)	10.8

Source: Survey data.

The details on storage and method of segregation of date expired drugs is presented in table 4.23. It can be seen from table that all the pharmacies ensured proper storage and segregation of date expired drugs. While for identifying expired medications in pharmacy, two third of pharmacist get alerts from computer and remaining one third of them regularly checks of medication. All pharmacist have reported that current procedures for managing expired medications in their pharmacy was separation of expired medicines and return to pharmaceutical distributor.

Table 4.23: Details on Storage and Method of Segregation of Date Expired Drugs

Sr. No.	***Particulars***	***Responses (%)***
1.	Do you (pharmacies) ensure proper storage and segregation of date expired drugs?	
	Yes	**100.0**
	No	**0.0**
2.	Current procedures for identifying expired medications in your pharmacy	
	(a) Regular checks of medication	33.33
	(b) Alerts from computer software	66.67
	(c) Brought to notice by Consumer	0.0
	(d) Any other	0.0
3.	Current procedures for managing expired medications in your pharmacy?	
	(a) Separation of expired medicines and Return to Pharmaceutical distributor	100.0
	(b) Separation of expired medicines and proper disposal of expired medicines	0.0
	(c) Incinerate through drug inspectorate	0.0
	(d) Dispose pf workplace garbage	0.0

The details on storage and method of segregation of date expired drugs are presented in Table 4.24. It can be seen from table that all the pharmacist reported that drug distributors or wholesalers collect back their date expired drugs and if needed, they dispose of expired drugs safely, without harming people or the environment (as per stipulated guidelines). Around 93 per cent pharmacists educate customers about the proper disposal of expired medicines. Around two third of pharmacists have policy to take back unused drugs from consumers. All pharmacists have reported that consumer check the expiry date on medicine while purchasing/taking to home.

Table 4.24: Details on Policy of Taking Back Unused Medicines

Sr. No.	*Particulars*	*(%)*
1.	Should drug distributors or wholesalers collect back their date expired drugs?	
	Yes	100.0
	No	0.0
2.	Have you dispose of expired drugs safely, without harming people or the environment (as per stipulated guidelines)	
	Yes	100.0
	No	0.0
3.	Do you educate customers about the proper disposal of expired medicines?	
	Yes	93.33
	No	6.67
4.	Do you have policy to take back unused drugs from consumers?	
	Yes	66.67
	No	33.33
5.	If yes, How many consumers generally return unused drugs in a month? (out of 100, how many return)	
6.	Does consumer check the expiry date on medicine while purchasing/taking to home?	
	Yes	100.0
	No	0.0
7.	If yes, how many consumers generally check expiry date while taking medicine to home? (out of 100, how many return)	39.55

The details on purchase and return of medicine behaviour of consumer reported by pharmacist are presented in Table 4.25 and observed that out of 100 consumers, 59% consumers buy medicine as per prescription, 23 per cent consumers buy medicine as per their own knowledge and 16 per cent consumers buy medicine as per advice of pharmacist.

Table 4.25: Medicine Purchase behaviour of Consumer

Sr. No.	*Particulars*	*(%)*
1.	How many consumers buy medicine as per prescription (out of 100)	58.67
2.	How many consumers buy medicine as per their own knowledge (out of 100)	25.33
3.	How many consumers buy medicine as per your advice (out of 100)	16.00

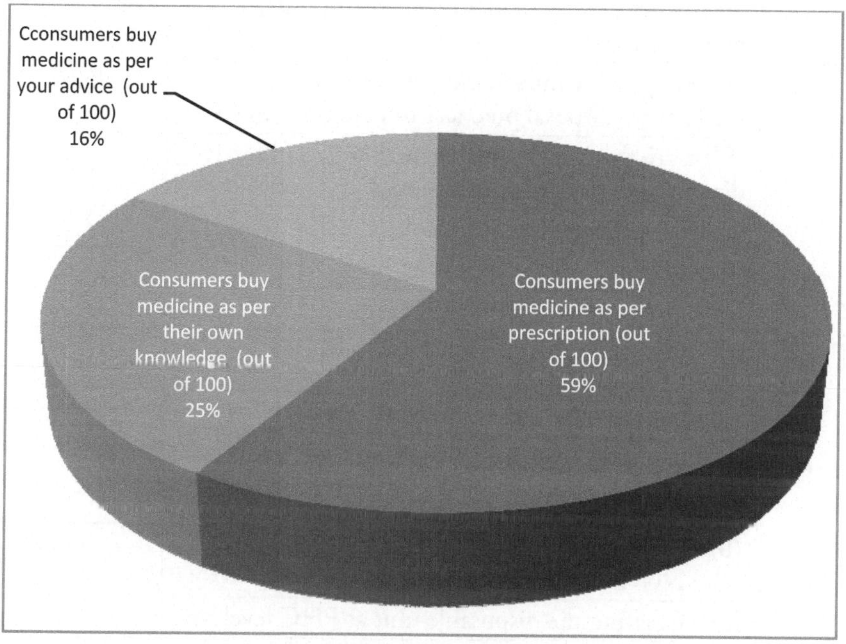

Figure 4.29: Purchase of Medicine behaviour of Consumer

Around 13.33 per cent consumers ask pharmacists about procedure to dispose-off date expired medicines, while 87 per cent of pharmacists provided information about proper medication disposal practices to patients. The biggest challenges pharmacists face in safely disposing of expired medications are Improper disposal practices (47%), Environ mental concerns (33%), Lack of standard protocols and Lack of trained personal (13%). All the pharmacists opined that massive awareness programs for consumers was suggested to enhance the safe disposal of expired medicines, while 7 per cent suggested to create the disposable unit at PHC level. All pharmacists suggested for a need for creating the awareness among consumers about drug disposal policy in India. For proper disposal of unused and date expired medicine, all pharmacists suggested to educate patients on how to dispose of medications safely. Around 13 per cent suggested to create programs to collect unwanted drugs from pharmacies.

Table 4.26: Details on Disposal of Medicine

Sr. No.	***Particulars***	***Responses (%)***
1.	How many consumers ask you about procedure to dispose off date expired medicines? (out of 100, how many)	13.00
2.	Do you provide information about proper medication disposal practices to patients? Yes (%)	86.67
3.	What are the biggest challenges you face in safely disposing of expired medications?	
	(a) Lack of standard protocols	13.33
	(b) Improper disposal practices	46.67
	(c) Environmental concerns	33.00
	(d) Lack of trained personal	13.33
	(e) Financial constraints	0.00
4.	What changes or improvements would you suggest to enhance the safe disposal of expired medicines?	
	(a) Massive awareness programs for consumers	100.00
	(b) Collection of unused medicines by some NGOs for further used	0.00
	(c) Creating the disposable unit at PHC level	6.67
5.	Is there a need for creating the awareness among consumers about drug disposal policy in India? Yes	100.00
6.	What are your recommendations for proper disposal of unused and date expired medicine?	
	(a) Educate patients on how to dispose of medications safely	100.0
	(b) Create standard protocols for disposing of expired medications	33.3
	(c) Create legislation to monitor and control the disposal of unused and expired medications	0.0
	(d) Create programs to collect unwanted drugs from pharmacies	13.33

4.4 Summary

The chapter presented the results of survey conducted and discussed the aspects related to use, storage and disposal of medicine.

The next chapter present the conclusion and policy implications.

CHAPTER V

Summary and Conclusions

5.1 Backdrop

Medicine consumption is increasing day by day all over the world, especially in countries like India and China. Global use of medicines grew by 14 per cent over the past five years (2020–2024) and a further 12 per cent increase is expected through 2028, bringing annual use to 3.8 trillion defined daily doses (GUM, 2024). The highest volume growth over the next five years is expected in China, India and Asia-Pacific, all exceeding 3 per cent compound annual growth. The coronavirus pandemic has increased prescription drug use and impacted the way people get their medications. India's pharmaceutical industry is the third largest by volume after China and Italy. While irrational use of medicines (overuse, underuse or misuse of medicines) results in wastage of scarce resources and widespread health hazards. is a major problem worldwide.

Though more emphasis is made on the rational use of medicine such that patients should receive the right medicines at the right time and use them appropriately. Most of the times these prescribed medicines are left unused due to various reasons like the change of treatment, side effects of the drug, improvement of patient condition resulting in discontinuation of the course of treatment. Re-use of leftover drugs for self-medication is unsafe which should be used only under the supervision of medical professional especially antibiotics and other prescription drugs. In addition, storage of unused medicine at home may increase the risk of a wide range of potential drug-related problems like errors in taking medications, adverse drug reactions, and can be considered as a waste of resources. Eventually these medicines are disposed off but there is a lacuna in proper disposal practices. Improper disposal of medicines can cause an environmental contamination which leads to health hazards. Currently, a high amount of pharmaceutical wastes flows through sewerage into the water bodies alarming the environmental scientist around the world and are also getting absorbed into the land when they are disposed of as solid waste in landfills. It was established that tons of municipal solid waste are generated due to expired and unused drugs. These are due to the improper disposal of unused medications through environmentally-unfriendly routes. To overcome this problem the proper handling of the expired drugs is imperative. Moreover, the improper drug disposal causes various consequences like accidental consumption of expired drugs, resale or misuse during sorting. The common preventive step to protect the environment from this kind of pharmaceutical waste is by creating the awareness about proper disposal method to avoid the pollution of environment and their impacts.

Unused and expired medicines are potentially toxic substances that should be managed effectively to avoid possible environmental hazards. The absence of well-defined protocols in India regarding the proper disposal of unused, unwanted, and expired medications raises concerns about the potential for accidental poisoning and environmental threats. The accumulation of unused and expired medicines in households and their disposal practices are serious global challenges that need to be investigated. India continues to have the persisting environmental problem of disposal of expired, unused, unwanted medicines. Since this has not been studied well, the exact repercussions, therefore, are not hitherto known fully. There has been no study regarding the disposal practices of unwanted pharmaceutical products conducted in Gujarat. The results of these studies are necessary for developing effective measures to increase public awareness of medication disposal and the harms associated with its improper practices. Although the National Formulary of India (2016 and 2021), specifies guidelines for the proper disposal of medicines, yet most of the people are not aware of these guidelines and the importance to follow them. As this is an emerging issue of concern, the present study was planned to carry out in Gujarat to address some of the questions pertaining to the disposal of unused pharmaceuticals by households and individuals include: what are the current methods employed by individuals to dispose of unused and expired pharmaceuticals?, Is their choice of disposal methods influenced by any prior knowledge of environmental issues associated with pharmaceuticals?; Most importantly, is there a need for a formalized protocol for disposal and destruction of unused and expired medications worldwide in order to minimize their potential impact on the global environment?. The data were collected by survey method from sample of 385 respondents three four categories was selected.(Pharmacy, Nursing, Bachelor of Education & Others) and fifteen registered pharmacies of the city located in and around the study area were also included in this study.

5.2 Findings from Survey Data

Profile of Selected Respondents

- The half of the selected respondents belongs to rural areas and rest half of respondents were from urban (semi-urban and urban area) in Gujarat.
- Out of the total selected sample respondents, around 37 percent were students of pharmacy degree, 30 per cent were Trainee Teacher students, 26 per cent were nursing diploma students and rest were others (7%).
- The dominance of female respondents (63%) was observed having more than one third share of male respondents (37%) at the overall level. Across the locality, except in semi-urban where male respondents were higher than female, picture was same as noticed at overall level.
- The average age of respondents was estimated to be around 21 years ranging from 21–25 across the locality.
- While education level of respondents was around pursuing graduation level education.
- As it was expected more than 98 per cent of respondents had possessed android application based mobile phone which has all facility available including immediate search about the medicine, its uses as well as disposal mechanism as prescribed by the government. It means almost everyone has available source at their tip of figures to get information related to medicine.
- As focus of study was to get awareness about of about use and disposal of medicines from youth and younger personals, more than 90 per cent of respondents were unmarried and rest were married one. Some of the student who are married are perusing their education for brighter future.
- In terms of size of family, average size of estimated to be around 5.3 person which ranges from 4.9 to 5.5 persons. One third of respondents belong to below poverty line while rest were from above poverty line income group. The occupation of the respondents was mainly being in pursuing in education were students.
- At overall level, majority of respondents were from general category (39%) followed by respondents from other backward classes

(29%), and Schedules tribes and Scheduled Caste (15.8% each). Across the locality, almost same kind trend was observed. In fact, rural locality has found more proper representation of SC and ST contributing more than 41 per cent share in total number of respondents.

- While in case of distribution of respondent's households as per their income level category, two third of total respondents were from above poverty line (66.5%) and rest were from below poverty line category (33.5%). Around 86 percent of respondents from urban and semi-urban locality were from APL category, while dominance of BPL and other category was found dominant in rural locality (53%)

About Use of Medication

- In order to meet the frequent need of medicine and for regular prescribed use of medicine in case of nay diseases or illness, some medicines are always kept at the home. The results indicate that almost half of the respondents have mentioned that they keep medicine at home (always+ often), while around 34 per cent keep medicine at home sometimes, while around 15 per cent keep it on rare case and rest were not keeping same at home.
- Storage is crucial for the safety and quality of medicines. Around 80 per cent of respondents have reported storing medicine in cool places such living room and bedroom, while around 13 per cent store them in refrigerators and some of them store in locker and rest of them are not clearly known about storage of medicine.
- Selected respondents have mentioned that they have been storing medication away from moisture, light and high temperature as and when instructed by the pharmacist or doctor.
- Though it has been advocated that never give medicine to someone without their consent or try to force them to take it, sharing prescription drugs without the proper permit is absolutely illegal. It was observed that around 12.21 per cent of respondents always share their medicines with relatives or friends, while 6.23 per cent respondents do it often and 38 per cent of respondents do it sometimes.
- Checking the expiration date of medicine before purchasing is crucial for ensuring its safety and effectiveness, as using expired medication can be harmful or ineffective. Around 87 per cent of

selected respondents have reported that they check expiry date printed on medicine while purchasing it which is welcome to note. It has been also advocated that before administering any medication, it should always verify the expiry date to ensure patient safety and efficacy. Expired medications can become ineffective or even harmful due to degradation or bacterial growth. Around 81 percent of respondents have reported that they verify the expiry date on medicine before administering medication.

About Used and Expired Medication at Home

- At overall level, around 88 per cent of respondents have reported that purchased medicines are remaining unused at home. Across the locality, the highest numbers of respondents were observed in Semi-urban area (90%) followed by around 89 per cent respondents from rural area and the lowest number of respondents (86%) reported having medicine at the home.
- Around 68 per cent of respondents had painkiller tablets (Analgesic medicine) at their home as usual required medicine at home. Around 41 per cent of respondents reported having antibiotic tablets at the home. Antidiabetic and digestions (41% respondents) related tablets are also been among medicines remain at home. While few of them (18–19%) also had, power and liquid state medicine related to digestion was also been reported unused at home.
- Out of respondents those who have reported, the average number of unused medications stored in household are presented in around 66 per cent of respondents reported having 0 to 5 medicines at home while around 18 per cent respondents were having 6–10 medicines at home. It was very strange to note that around 9 per cent of respondents have reported having more than 20 medicine at home. Around 88 per cent of respondents have reported having prescribed medicine at the home while 42 percent of residents non-prescribed medicines at home. Thus, medicines have been kept at home of both the nature (prescribed and non-prescribed).
- In case of date expired medicines, as per responses received, around 89 per cent respondents have mentioned of having 0–5 date expired medicines, while hardly one per cent have reported having more than 20 date expired medicines. The medicines which was

date expired was mostly prescribed one (60%) followed by 29 per cent of non-prescribed medicines .

- Medicine use can be influenced by several factors. The major reason cited by the respondents for keeping purchased medicine unused at home was disease or condition got resolved or patient recovered (69%) followed by change of medication by the doctor (49%) and forgetting to take medicine (40%). While some of them have reported medicine due to experiencing side effect (33%) and bitter taste (36%). Around 31 per cent respondent reported that due to change of doctor or starting of another treatment, medicine remained unused.

Knowledge on Disposal of Unused and Expired Medication

- Around 64 per cent of respondents agreed that they are aware about the fact that misused/repeated change or not complete antibiotics may cause drug resistance. While 37 per cent respondents knew about "drug-take-back system.
- Around 67 percent of respondents separate unused medicine before disposal. While, in case of date expired medicines, 23-24 per cent respondents know about medication waste and they read medicines disposal instruction and they have you ever followed medicines disposal instruction. These respondents must have from the pharmaceutical and nursery diploma holders background who have received some information about the disposal of same.
- Around 67 per cent of respondents knew that improper disposal of unused and expired medicines can affect the environment and health. Only one third of them have reported receiving education regarding safe disposal of medication. Very few of them reported seeking information from official resources safe disposals of medications.
- Among the selected respondents' household, common disposal practices for unused and expired medicines include throwing them in the garbage/trash as reported by 74 per cent of respondents, while 27 per cent of respondents have disposed it by burning followed 22 per cent of respondents have flushed them down the toilet or sink. It indicates significant portion also unaware of proper disposal methods.
- In case of date-expired medicine disposal practises, around 76 per cent of respondents reported throwing them away in household

garbage followed by 22 per cent respondents flushing them in toilets. Around 27 per cent respondent mentioned that date-expired medicines were disposed by burning it.

- All the respondents agreed opined that unused medicines should not be thrown into dustbins and burning of expired medicines can release toxic substances which can be inhaled by the people. Also, all agreed for the fact that there should be a public awareness program about the harmful effects of improper medicine disposal practices.
- Around 97 percent of respondents opined that unsafe practices of medicines disposal can pollute the environment. Around 93 per cent of respondents agreed on the fact that community pharmacists have an important role in mitigating the problem of improper medicine disposal practices.

Actions to control the hazardous effect of unused and expired medicines

- Safely dispose of unused or expired medicines before they can do harm. There are many ways to get rid of them. The 72 per cent of respondents suggested to providing proper guidance to the consumer, while 63 per cent opined that same can be done consuming the same as per doctor advice.
- Around 60 per cent of respondents suggested to prescribe in quantities and for duration that ensure patient compliance while 55 per cent suggested to deposit unused medicine in nearby Public Health Centre.
- Around 39–41 per cent of respondents have suggested to donate the unused medicines and also by lowering the number of prescribed medicines by doctor.
- The respondents were asked to mentioned about their perception about bodies responsible for creation of awareness about disposal of unused and expired medication. The 61 per cent respondent opined that government mechanism (health department and related sections) followed by health bureau (57%) should create awareness about proper disposal of unused and expired medications. Around 55 per cent respondents noted that awareness need to be spearheaded by pharmacists followed by healthcare professionals, i.e. physician and doctors (50%).
- Around 87 per cent of respondents have suggested to arrange awareness program in every village/hospital, while around 65–67

percent of respondents opined to create awareness through print (newspaper/magazines), air and electronic media (Program on TV, Radio) and digital (Youtube, Facebook, Whatsup, instagram) media. While 61 per cent of respondents suggested to include topic on use and disposal pf medicine in school curriculum

- All the selected respondents perceived that there is a need for a program to collect unused medicines from home. All the selected respondents also agreed that consumers should be made more aware about donation of medicines and hazards of unsafe disposal & methods of safe disposal
- Around 55 percent of respondents have suggested to keep medicine at proper places followed by 35 percent respondents suggested to return unused medicine to chemist followed by 29 per cent respondents suggested to organise awareness programs at schools to improve awareness of consumers regarding safe disposal of medicines.

Response of Pharmacists

- Pharmacists are key players in the pharmaceutical supply chain and are in a position to contribute to the reduction of medication waste and for creating awareness about proper disposal of medicines by educating patients, participating in take-back programs, and implementing effective inventory management practices within pharmacies. The survey results indicate that majority of the pharmacist were from Urban area (53%) followed by semi urban (40%) and rest were from rural areas (table 4.22). All the pharmacists were registered drug shoppers. Around three fifth of
- Pharmacists possess diploma level of education while rest of two fifth were graduated in pharmacy/science subject. Out of total selected pharmacist, 73 per cent were male and rest were female respondents (27%). The average age of respondent pharmacist were estimated to be 34 years and having experience of around 11 years in pharmacy.
- All the pharmacies ensured proper storage and segregation of date expired drugs. While for identifying expired medications in pharmacy, two third of pharmacist get alerts from computer and remaining one third of them regularly checks of medication. All pharmacist have reported that current procedures for managing

expired medications in their pharmacy was separation of expired medicines and return to pharmaceutical distributor.

- All the pharmacist reported that drug distributors or wholesalers collect back their date expired drugs and if needed, they dispose of expired drugs safely, without harming people or the environment (as per stipulated guidelines). Around 93 per cent pharmacists educate customers about the proper disposal of expired medicines. Around two third of pharmacists have policy to take back unused drugs from consumers. All pharmacists have reported that consumer check the expiry date on medicine while purchasing/ taking to home.
- Out of 100 consumers, 59% consumers buy medicine as per prescription, 23 per cent consumers buy medicine as per their own knowledge and 16 per cent consumers buy medicine as per advice of pharmacist.
- Around 13.33 per cent consumers ask pharmacists about procedure to dispose-off date expired medicines, while 87 per cent of pharmacists provided information about proper medication disposal practices to patients.
- The biggest challenges pharmacists face in safely disposing of expired medications are Improper disposal practices (47%), Environmental concerns (33%), Lack of standard protocols and Lack of trained personal (13%). All the pharmacists opined that massive awareness programs for consumers was suggested to enhance the safe disposal of expired medicines, while 7 per cent suggested to create the disposable unit at PHC level. All pharmacists suggested for a need for creating the awareness among consumers about drug disposal policy in India.
- For proper disposal of unused and date expired medicine, all pharmacists suggested to educate patients on how to dispose of medications safely. Around 13 per cent suggested to create programs to collect unwanted drugs from pharmacies.

5.3 Conclusions

Our findings indicate that a majority of the participants tend to dispose of medicines in an unsafe manner. Conversely, the responsible disposal of medications is significantly influenced by patient education. Hence, healthcare professionals are better positioned to impart knowledge to the public, fostering awareness about the proper storage and safe disposal of unused, unwanted, and expired medicines. There is a need of the hour to take stringent actions and formulate uniform guidelines on the safe disposal of medicines. Moreover, safe disposal instructions should be provided by all healthcare providers to patients in routine practice. Thus, efforts need to be done by every section of the society for the safe disposal of medications in order to create a safe environment for future.

5.4 Policy Implications

The study brings out following policy implications:

- From the present study it can be concluded that the consumers had poor knowledge regarding the safe drug disposal techniques. Therefore, it is the need of the hour to take stringent actions and formulate uniform guidelines on the safe disposal of medicines. Moreover, safe disposal instructions should be provided by all healthcare providers to patients in routine practice. Thus, efforts need to be done by every section of the society for the safe disposal of medications in order to create a safe environment for future.
- Awareness program should be conducted periodically to all the healthcare professionals to practice as well as advice and motivate the general public on safe drug disposal. Media like television, social networks should be used to propagate the challenges to the environment due to improper disposal drugs of the disposal
- There is a need of drug take back program. A take back program will provide timely disposal methods and may lessen likelihood of medication waste going through the sewage system, and hence environmental pollution may be prevented. Government should implement a national level drug take back program preferably collecting the returned unused or expired drugs at every level of Government hospitals. Residents need to be inform to return undesired prescriptions to pharmacies, which are then collected and destroyed by approved agents or bodies
- The medicine takeback system can be initially implemented in community pharmacies located in major cities and information about the system be widely disseminated.
- Strict legal framework, well organized, cost-effective and easily accessible state-run disposal systems are necessary in order to enable the general public to reduce negative pharmaceutical

impacts on the environment by returning unused pharmaceuticals to collection schemes for proper disposal.

- There is a need to include topic on proper use, storage and disposal of medicine in school curriculum.

References

Abahussain, E., Waheedi, M. and Koshy, S. (2012). Practice, awareness and opinion of pharmacists toward disposal of unwanted medications in Kuwait. *Saudi Pharmaceutical Journal,* 20(3):195–201.

Abahussain, E.A. and Ball, D.E. (2007). Disposal of unwanted medicines from households in Kuwait, 29(4):368–373.

Abahussain, E.A., Ball, D.E. and Matowe, W.C. (2006). Practice and opinion towards disposal of unused medication in Kuwait. *Med Princ Pract,* 15(5):352–7.

Abdallah, Q.M.A., Al-Haddad, M.S.M., Al-Khathami, O.H.M., Al-Kherish, O.H.H., Al-Marri, K.M.T. and Al-Matani, M.F.K., *et al.* (2014). Knowledge, attitude and practice towards discarding unwanted household medicines among university students in Western region, KSA. *Int J Pharm,* 4(4):14–21.

Abdi, A., Faraji, A., Dehghan, F. and Khatony, A. (2018). Prevalence of self-medication practice among health sciences students in Kermanshah, Iran. *BMC Pharmacol Toxicol.* 2018 Jul 3; 19(1):36. doi: 10.1186/s40 360-018-0231-4. PMID: 29970167; PMCID: PMC6029137.

Abdo-Rabbo, A., Al-Ansari, M., Gunn, B.C. and Suleiman, B.J. (2009). The use of medicines in Oman. *Sultan Qaboos Univ Med J.* 9(2):124–131.

Abou-Auda, H.S. (2003). An economic assessment of the extent of medication use and wastage among families in Saudi Arabia and Arabian Gulf countries. *Clin Ther* 25(4):1276–1292.

Abrous, J., Vadala, T., Miller, S. and Cerulli, J. (2010). Encouraging safe medication disposal through student pharmacist intervention. *J Am Pharm Assoc.,* 50:169–173.

Aditya, S. and Singh, H. (2013). Safe medication disposal: Need to sensitize undergraduate students. *International Journal of Pharmacy & Life Sciences.* 4(3), 2475–80.

Ahmed, A. and Mushtaq, N. (2013). Disposal practices of unused and expired pharmaceuticals in Karachi and their impact on health and environment. *Journal of University Medical & Dental College,* 2013; 4(2):42–48.

Alghadeer, S. and Al-Arifi, M.N. (2021). Community pharmacists' practice, awareness, and beliefs about drug disposal in Saudi Arabia. *Healthcare. MDPI;* 9(7):823.

Alhomoud, F.K., Alsadiq, Y., Alghalawin, L., Alhifany, A. and Alhomoud, F. (2020). Pharmacy students' knowledge and practices concerning the storing and disposal of household medication in Saudi Arabia. *Curr*

Pharm Teach Learn. 2021 Jan; 13(1):5–13. doi: 10.1016/j.cptl.2020.08.004. Epub 2020 Aug 25. PMID: 33131618.

Al-Maaded, M., Madi, N.K., Kahraman, R., Hodzic, A. and Ozerkan, N.G. (2012) An overview of solid waste management and plastic recycling in Qatar. J Polym Environ 20(1):186–194.

Al-Shareef, F., El-Asrar, S.A., Al-Bakr, L., Al-Amro, M., Alqahtani, F., Aleanizy, F. and Al-Rashood, S. (2016). Investigating the disposal of expired and unused medication in Riyadh, Saudi Arabia: A cross-sectional study. *Int. J. Clin Pharm,* 6; 38(4):822–8.

Alshehri, Deemah and Haneen, Banjar (2021). Increasing Awareness of Proper Disposal of Unused and Expired Medication Using a Knowledge-Based Disposal Management System, *Journal of Environmental and Public Health* Volume 10.

Althagafia, Abdulhamid; Mohannad, Alshibania; Samah, Alshehria; Ahmed, Noora; Alaa, Baglagela and Tahani, Almeleebiac (2022). Assessment of knowledge and awareness of safe disposal of unused or expired medication in Saudi Arabia: A cross-sectional study, *Saudi Pharmaceutical Journal,* 30, 1672–1678.

Angi'enda, S.A. and Bukachi, S.A. (2016). Household knowledge and perceptions on disposal practices of unused medicines in Kenya. *Journal of Anthropological Archaeology,* 4(2):1–20.

Arkaravichien, W., Ruchipiyarak, T., Thawinwan, W. and Benjawilaikul, S. (2014). A threat to the environment from practice of drug disposal in Thailand. *Environ Asia,* 7(1):13–8.

Aryal, A., Anuba, P.A., Arun, G.R., Sarumathy, S. and Kumar, R.N. (2023). A review on status of drug disposal practice of unused and expired drugs among different countries. *J Appl Pharm Sci,* 2023; 13(04):045–052. https://doi.org/10.7324/JAPS.2023.32158

Aryal, A., Anuba, P.A., Arun, G.R, Sarumathy, S. and Kumar, R.N. A review on status of drug disposal practice of unused and expired drugs among different countries. *J Appl Pharm Sci,* 2023; 13(04):045–052.

Atinafu, T., Takele, A., Kassie, A., Yehualaw, A., Tesfaw, G. and Desseno, T., *et al.* (2014). Unused medications disposal practice: The case of Patients visiting university of Gondar specialized teaching Hospital, Gondar, *Ethiopia. Int J Pharm Sci Res.* 2014; 5(12): 999–1005.

Aukidy Al, M., Verlicchi, P., Jelic, A., Petrovic, M. and Barcel, D. Barcel (2012). Monitoring release of pharmaceutical compounds: occurrence and environmental risk assessment of two WWTP effluents and their receiving bodies in the Po Valley, Italy. *Sci Total Environ.* 2012; 438:15–25. DOI: 10.1016/j.scitotenv.2012.08.061

Auta, A., Banwat, S.B., Sariem, C.N., Shalkur, D., Nasara, B. and Atuluku, M.O. (2012). Medicines in pharmacy students' residence and self-medication practices. *J Young Pharm,* 4(2):119–23.

Auta, A., Banwat, S., Sariem, C., Shalkur, D., Nasara, B. and Atuluku, M. (2012) Medicines in pharmacy students' residence and self-medication practices. *J Young Pharm,* 4(2):119–123.

Auta, A., Omale, S., Shalkur, D. and Abiodun, A.H. (2011) Unused medicines in Nigerian households: types and disposal practices. *J. Pharmacol Pharmacother,* 2(3):195–196

Ayele, Y. and Mamu, M. (2018). Assessment of knowledge, attitude and practice towards disposal of unused and expired pharmaceuticals among community in Harar city, Eastern Ethiopia. *Journal of Pharmaceutical Policy and Practice,* 11(1):27.

Azmi Hassali, M., Shakeel, S. (2020). Unused and expired medications disposal practices among the general public in Selangor, Malaysia. *Pharmacy,* 2020; 8(4):196.

Barnett-Itzhaki, Z., Berman, T., Grotto, I. and Schwartzberg, E. (2016). Household medical waste disposal policy in Israel. *Isr J Health Policy Res,* 5, p. 48, 10.1186/s13584-016-0108-1

Bashaar, M. Mohammadl; Vijay, Thawani; Mohamed, Azmi Hassali and Fahad, Saleem (2017). Disposal practices of unused and expired pharmaceuticals among general public in Kabul. *BMC Public Health,* 2017; 17(1):45. https://doi.org/10.1186/s12889-016-3975-z.

Bashatah, A. and Wajid, S. (2020). Knowledge and disposal practice of Leftover and Expired Medicine: a cross-sectional study from nursing and pharmacy students' perspectives. *Int J Environ Res Public Health,* 2020; 17(6):2068. https://doi. org/10.3390/ijerph17062068.

Begum, M.M., Rivu, S.F., Hasan, M.M.A., Nova, T.T., Rahman, M.M., Alim, M.A., Uddin, M.S., Islam, A., Nurnahar, Tabassum, N., Moni, M.M.R., Roselin, R., Das, M., Begum, R. and Rahman, M.S. (2021). Disposal Practices of Unused and Leftover Medicines in the Households of Dhaka Metropolis. *Pharmacy, 9*(2), 103.

Bhaiya, R. (n.d). Community Based Solid Waste Management Through Public-Private-Community Partnerships: Experience of Waste Concern in Bangladesh.

Borhan Uddin, M., Al Samir, R. and Golam Mehebub Pantho, G.M. (2024). Practice of Expired and Unused Drug Disposal in South Asian and Southeast Asian Countries. *IntechOpen.* doi: 10.5772/intechopen. 1006861

Bound, J., Kitsou, K. and Voulvoulis, N. (2006). Household disposal of pharmaceuticals and the perception of risk to the environment. *Environ Toxicol Pharmacol* 21:301–307.

Bound, J.P. and Voulvoulis, N. (2005). Household disposal of pharmaceuticals as a pathway for aquatic contamination in the United Kingdom. *Environmental health perspectives.* 2005 Dec; 113(12):1705.

Braund, R., Peake, B. and Shieffelbien, L. (2009) Disposal practices for unused medications in New Zealand. *Environ Int* 35:952–955.

Bungau, S., Tit, D.M., Fodor, K., Cioca, G., Agop, M., Iovan, C., Cseppento, D.C.N., Bumbu, A. and Bustea, C. (2008). Aspects regarding the pharmaceutical waste management in Romania. *Sustainability*, 10(8):2788.

Chartier, Y. (Ed.). (2014). *Safe management of wastes from health-care activities*. World Health Organization.

Chaturvedi, Preeti; Parul, Shukla; Balendu, Shekher Giri; Pankaj, Chowdhary; Ram, Chandra; Pratima, Gupta and Ashok, Pandey (2021). Prevalence and hazardous impact of pharmaceutical and personal care products and antibiotics in environment: A review on emerging contaminants, *Environmental Research*, Volume 194, https://doi.org/10.1016/j.envres.2020.110664.

Coma, A., Modamio, P., Lastra, C.F., Bouvy, M.L. and Mariño, E.L. (2008). Returned medicines in community pharmacies of Barcelona, Spain. *Pharm World Sci*; 30(3):272–7.

Dar, M.A., Maqbool, M. and Rasool, S. (2019). Pharmaceutical wastes and their disposal practice in routine. *Int J Inf Comput Sci*, *6*, 76–92.

Daughton, C.G., Ternes, T.A. (1999). Pharmaceuticals and personal care products in the environment: agents of subtle change? *Environ Health Perspect*, 1999; 107(6):907–38.

Directive 1999/31/EC of the European Parliament and of the Council of 26 April 1999 on the landfill of waste, *Official Journal* L—182, 17 July 1999, p. 1–19.

Directive 2001/83/EC of the European Parliament and of the Council of 6 November 2001 on the community code relating to medicinal products for human use. *Official Journal* L–311, 28 Nov. 2001, p. 67–128, article 127.

Directive 2004/27/EC of the European Parliament and of the Council of 31 March 2004 amending 2001/83/EC on the community code relating to medicinal products for human use. *Official Journal* L—136, 30 Apr 2004, p. 57, article 127b.

Donatini, A. (2019). International Health Care System Profiles. Italy : International health care system profiles. [Cited 2019 Sep. 29]. Available from: https://international.commonwealthfund.org/countries/italy.

Ehrhart, Amy L. Elise, F. Granek, Max Nielsen-Pincus and Dorothy A. Horn (2020). Leftover drug disposal: Customer behavior, pharmacist recommendations, and obstacles to drug take-back box implementation, Waste Management, Volume 118, 2020, 416–425 (https://doi.org/10.1016/j.wasman.2020.08.038).

FDA (2013). Where and How to Dispose of Unused Medicines. Available at: www.fda.gov/ForConsumers/ConsumerUpdates/ucm101653.htm. Accessed 5 November 2013.

Fenech, C., Rock, L., Nolan, K. and Morrissey, A. (2013). Attitudes towards the use and disposal of unused medications in two European Countries. *Waste Manag* 33(2):259–261.

Gotz, K. and Keil, F. (2007). Drug disposal in private households: does the disposal of pharmaceuticals via domestic sanitary devices contribute to water contamination? Z Umweltchem Okotox 19:180–188

Government of India (2011). National Formulary of India, 2011. Ministry of Health and Family Welfare. Available at: https://Www.Nhp.Gov.In/National-Formulary-Of-India_Mtl.

GUM (2024). Global Use of Medicine 2024–Outlook to 2028, Retrieved from https://www.iqvia.com/insights/the-iqvia-institute/reports-and-publications/reports/the-global-use-of-medicines-2024.

Gupta, D., Gupta, A., Ansari, N.A. and Ahmed, O.S. (2013). Patient's opinion and practice towards unused medication disposal: A qualitative study. *J Pharm Sci Innov.*, 2:47–50.

Gupta, Rohini, Gupta B.M. and Gupta, Apeksha (2018). A study on awareness regarding disposal of unused medicines among consumers ar a tertiary care teaching hospital of North India. *International Journal of Advances in Medicines*, 91–95.

Labu, K.Z., Al-Mamun, M.M.A., Harun, M. and Sikder, K. (2013). Knowledge, awareness and disposal practice for unused medications among the students of the Private University of Bangladesh. *J. Biomed Pharm Res* 2(2):26–33.

Insani, W.N., Qonita, N.A., Jannah, S.S., Nuraliyah, N.M., Supadmi, W., Gatera, V.A., Alfian, S.D. and Abdulah, R. (2020). Improper disposal practice of unused and expired pharmaceutical products in Indonesian households. *Heliyon*, 2020 Jul 29; 6(7):e04551. doi: 10.1016/j.heliyon.2020.e04551. PMID: 32760838; PMCID: PMC7393449.

Jha, Nisha; Sajala, Kafle; Shital, Bhandary and Pathiyil, Ravi Shankar (2022). Assessment of Knowledge, Attitude, and Practise of disposing and storing unused and expired medicines among the communities of Kathmandu, *Nepal, PLoS One,* 17 (8):e0272635.Raja

JPMA (2018). Japan Pharmaceutical Manufacturers Association. Procedures for disposal of medical and pharmaceutical product containers/packaging. February 2007. [Cited 2019 Sep 20] Available from: http://www.isoki.net/k2hirosakiyaku/pdf_folder/ 2008.07.10.pdf.

Kahsay, Halefom; Ahmedin, Mubarek; Binyam, Kebede; Kilay, Gebrezihar; Haylay, Araya and Desta, Tesfay (2020). Assessment of Knowledge, Attitude, and Expired Pharmaceuticals in Community of Adigrat City,

Northern Ethiopia. *Journal of Environmental and Public Health*, 6725423, 1–11.

Kaladharan, Sanju; Dhanya, M. and Rejikumar, G. (2023). Household Pharmaceutical Disposal Practices in India. *Economic and Politica Wekle*, Vol. 58, Issue No. 11, 18.

Kamal, K.M., Chiumente, M., Nakagawa, S., Giannetti, V. and Marlin, T. (2022). Disposal practices for unused and expired medications: pilot data from three cities in three countries. *GMS Health Innov Technol.* Mar 7; 16: Doc01. doi: 10.3205/hta000133. PMID: 35360086; PMCID: PMC8953661.

Kanyari, S.S., Senapati, T.R. and Kar, A. (2024). Disposal Practices of Unused and Expired Medicines Among the General Public and Pharmacies: A Mixed-Method Study in the Odisha State of Eastern India. *Cureus*. 2024 Jan 16; 16(1):e52359. doi: 10.7759/cureus.52359. PMID: 38361720; PMCID: PMC10867696.

Khan, U., Bloom, R., Nicell, J. and Laurenson, J. (2017). Risks associated with the environmental release of pharmaceuticals on the U.S. Food and Drug Administration flush list. *Sci Total Environ.* 2017; 609:1023–40. DOI: 0.1016/j.scitotenv.2017.05.269 12.

Kheir, N., Hajj, M.S., Wilbur, K. and Kaissi, R.M.L. (2011) An exploratory study on medications in Qatar homes. *Drug Healthc Patient Saf* 3:99–106.

Köksoy, S. (2024). Unused, expired pharmaceuticals and their disposal practices among the general public in Burdur-Türkiye: A cross-sectional study. BMC Public Health. 2024 May 13; 24(1):1303. doi: 10.1186/s12889-024-18788-0. PMID: 38741105; PMCID: PMC11092099.

Kotchen, M., Kallaos, J., Wheeler, K., Wong, C. and Zahller, M. (2009) Pharmaceuticals in wastewater: behaviour, preferences, and willingness to pay for a disposal program. *J Environ Manage* 90:1476–1482

Kozak, M.A., Melton, J.R., Gernant, S.A. and Snyder, M.E. (2016). A needs assessment of unused and expired medication disposal practices: a study from the Medication Safety Research Network of Indiana. *Res Social Adm Pharm,* 12(2):336–40.

Kruopiene,˙ J. and Dvarioniene,˙J. (2010) Management of environmental risks in the life cycle of human pharmaceuticals in Lithuania. *Environ Res Eng Manage* 2(52):41–47.

Krupiene, J. and Dvarioniene, J. (2007) Pharmaceutical pathways to the environment in Lithuania. *Environ Res Eng Manage* 41:33–39.

Kusturica, M.P., Sabo, A., Tomic, Z., Horvat, O. and Sˇolak, Z. (2012) Storage and disposal of unused medications: knowledge, behavior, and attitudes among Serbian people. *Int J Clin Pharm* 34:604–610.

Labu, Z.K. and Harun-Or-Rashid, M. (2016). Evaluation of safe disposal practice of unused medications among the students of world university of Bangladesh (WUB). *South Asian J. Popul Health*, 9(1) 45–55.

Law, A.V., Sakharkar, P., Zargarzadeh, A., Tai, B.W., Hess, K., Hata, M., Mireles, R., Ha, C. and Park, T.J. (2014) Taking stock of medication wastage: unused medications in US households. *Res Social Adm Pharm* 11(4):571–578.

Law, A.V., Sakharkar, P., Zargarzadeh, A., Tai, B.W., Hess, K. and Hata, M. (2015). Taking stock of medication wastage: Unused medications in US households. *Res Social Admin Pharm.* 2015; 11(4):571 78. DOI: 10.1016/j.sapharm.2014.10.003

Lewis, E.T., Cucciare, M.A. and Trafton, J.A. (2014). What do patients do with unused opioid medications? *Clin J Pain.* 2014; 30(8):654–62. DOI: 10.1097/ 01.ajp.0000435447.96642.f4

Manocha, S., Suranagi, U.D., Sah, R.K., Chandane, R.D., Kulhare, S., Goyal, N. and Tanwar, K. (2020). Current Disposal Practices of Unused and Expired Medicines Among General Public in Delhi and National Capital Region, India. Curr Drug Saf. 2020; 15(1):13–19. doi: 10.2174/1574886314666191008095344. PMID: 31593533.

Masoner, J.R., Kolpin, D.W., Furlong, E.T., Cozzarelli, I.M., Gray, J.L. and Schwab, E.A. (2014) Contaminants of emerging concern in fresh leachate from landfills in the conterminous United States. *Environ Sci Process Impacts* 16(10):2335–2354.

Matson, K.L., Pawsauskas, J.E. and Procopio, F. (2015). Reported behaviors of prescription-drug misuse and medication safety among students attending a Rhode Island university. *R I Med J.* 2015; 98(6):37 40.

Maughan, B.C., Hersh, E.V., Shofer, F.S., Wanner, K.J., Archer, E. and Carrasco, L.R. (2016). Unused opioid analgesics and drug disposal following outpatient dental surgery: A randomized controlled trial. *Drug Alcohol Depend.* 168:328–34. DOI: 10.1016/j.drugalcdep.2016.08.016

Medhi, B. and Sewal, R.K. (2012). Ecopharma covigilance: an issue urgently to be addressed. *Indian J Pharmacol,* 44(5):547–9.

Michael, I., Ogbonna, B., Sunday, N., Anetoh, M. and Matthew, O. (2019). Assessment of disposal practices of expired and unused medications among community pharmacies in Anambra state Southeast Nigeria: a mixed study design. *J Pharm Policy Pract*, 12 (2019), p. 12, 10.1186/s40545-019-0174-1.

Muhammad, Shoaib; Abdul, Raziq; Qaiser, Iqbal; Fahad, Saleem; Sajjad, Haider; Rabia, Ishaq; Zaffar, Iqbal and Mohammad, Bashaar (2022). Disposal practices of unused and expired pharmaceuticals among the general public in Quetta city, Pakistan. PLoS ONE. 2022; 17(5):e0268200. https://doi.org/10.1371/journal.pone.0268200.

Naser, A.Y., Amara, N., Dagash, A. and Naddaf, A. (2021). Medications disposal and medications storage in Jordan: A cross-sectional study. *International Journal of Clinical Practice*, *75*(3), e13822.

Nishibata, Y., Obata, H., Kimura, T., Jyounou, I., Takahashi, Y. and Tsukishima, S. (2019). Academic Committee Second Academic Subcommittee Report (Final Report) Investigation of disposal strategies for packaging/containers of medical and pharmaceutical products. *J Jpn Soc Hosp Pharm.*, 38(8), 1007 13. [Cited 2019 Sep 20] Available from: https://jshp.or.jp/gakujyutu/houkoku/h13gaku2.pdf 20.

OECD (2021). Health at a Glance 2021: OECD Indicators, Health at a Glance. doi:10.1787/ae3016b9-en

Orok, E., Erah, P. and Toe, J. Assessment of knowledge, awareness and disposal practices of unused and expired household medicines in the Parker Corner Road Community in Liberia. Research Square; 2023. DOI: 10.21203/rs.3.rs-2574947/v1.

Pankajkumar, P., Chacko, S., Res BP-JP. Storage and disposal of medicines in home among students. *J Pharm Res*, 2016; 10(6):343–50.

Paut Kusturica, Milica & Tomas Petrovic, Ana and Sabo, Ana. (2016). Disposal of Unused Drugs: Knowledge and Behavior Among People Around the World. *Reviews of Environmental Contamination and Toxicology*, Volume 240, 10.1007/398_2016_3.

Persson, M., Sabelstr om, E. and Gunnarsson, B. (2009) Handling of unused prescription drugs- knowledge, behaviour and attitude among Swedish people. *Environ Int* 35:771–774.

Persson, M., Sabelström, E. and Gunnarsson, B. (2009). Handling of unused prescription drugs—knowledge, behaviour and attitude among Swedish people. *Environment international*, *35*(5), 771–774.

Prakash, D., Sudhakaran, S. and Shabaraya, A.R. (2020). Global Scenario of Drug Disposal: A Review of Literature. *J Basic Clin Pharma*. 11:01–04.

Prinja, S., Kumar, S., Sharma, A., Kar, S.S., Tripathi, N., Dumka, N., Sharma, S., Mukhopadhyay, I., Rana, S.K., Garg, S., Kotwal, A. and Aggarwal, A.K. (2022). What is the out-of-pocket expenditure on medicines in India? An empirical assessment using a novel methodology. *Health Policy Plan*, 2022 Oct 12; 37(9):1116–1128. doi: 10.1093/heapol/czac057. PMID: 35862250.

Raja, S., Mohapatra, S., Ramu, T. and Rani, J. (2022). Knowledge, Attitude and Practice (KAP) Towards Disposal of Unused and Expired Medications: an Assessment Among Patients. *Biomed Pharmacol Journal*, 15(3).

Raja, Sangeetha; Satyajit, Mohapatra; Kalaiselvi, A. and Rani, R. Jamuna (2018). Awareness and Disposal Practices of Unused and Expired Medication among Health Care Professionals and Students in a Tertiary Care Teaching Hospital. *Biomedical & Pharmacology Journal*, Vol. 11(4), p. 2073–2078.

Reddy, A., De la Cruz, M., Rodriguez, E.M., Thames, J., Wu, J., Chisholm, G. and Liu, D. *et al.* (2014). Patterns of storage, use, and disposal of opioids among cancer outpatients. *Oncologist* 19:780–785.

Roy, V., Gupta, U. and Agarwal, A.K. (2012). Cost of medicines & their affordability in private pharmacies in Delhi (India). *Indian J Med Res.* 2012 Nov; 136(5):827–35. PMID: 23287131; PMCID: PMC3573605.

Ruhoy, I.S., Daughton Bound, J.P. and Voulvoulis, N. (2005) Household disposal of pharmaceuticals as a pathway for aquatic contamination in the United Kingdom. *Environ Health Perspect.* 2005; 113(12):1705–11. 11.

Ruhoy, I.S. and Daughton, C.G. (2007). Types and quantities of leftover drugs entering the environment via disposal to sewage—revealed by Coroner Records. *Sci Total Environ* 388(1–3):137–148.

Sarraf, D., Rauniar, G., Kushwaha, R., Keshwar, S. and Maharjan, R. (2022). Knowledge, attitude and practice of disposal of unused, unwanted and expired medicines among healthcare professionals. *Kathmandu University Medical Journal*, 2022; 20(3):323–329.

Sarraf, D., Rauniar, G., Kushwaha, R., Keshwar, S. and Maharjan, R. (2022). Knowledge, attitude and practice of disposal of unused, unwanted and expired medicines among healthcare professionals. *Kathmandu University Medical Journal* 20(3):323–329.

Sasu, S., K ummerer, K. and Kranert, M. (2012). Assessment of pharmaceutical waste management at selected hospitals and homes in Ghana. *Waste Manag Res* 30(6):625–630.

Seehusen, D.A. and Edwards, J. (2006). Patient practices and beliefs concerning disposal of medications. *J Am Board Family Med.* Nov 1; 19(6):542–7.

Sharma, A.; Ankush, Madaan and Anantha, Naik Nagappa (2012). Medication storage and self medication practice among the youth in Karnataka Region, *India. Int J Pharm Sci Res*, 3(8):2795–800.

Shivaraju, P.T. and Gangadhar, M. (2017). Knowledge and awareness of disposal of unused and expired medications among medical undergraduates of A Tertiary Care Teaching Hospital at BG Nagar: A cross-sectional observational study. *Natl J. Physiol Pharm Pharmacol* 2017; 7(11):1268–1273.

Shoaib, M., Raziq, A., Iqbal, Q., Saleem, F., Haider, S. and Ishaq, R., *et al.* (2022). Disposal practices of unused and expired pharmaceuticals among the general public in Quetta city, Pakistan. PLoS ONE 17(5): e0268200.

Shwetha, N. and Jha, A. (2018). Knowledge and awareness regarding safe drug disposal system among general population of India. *Journal of Pharmacovigilance,* 6(2):256.

Sirisha, A., Janardhan, M., Sree, P.K., Rao, Y.V., Raikar, S.R. and Patil, S. (2016). Knowledge, attitude and practice on safe disposal of medicines among medical and dental undergraduates. *J Basic Clin Res.* 3(1):5–9.

Swaroop, H.S., Charaborty, A. and Virupakshaiah, A. (2015). Knowledge, attitude and practice of medical professionals towards the safe disposal of unused medications in South India. *World J Pharm Pharm Sci.* 2015 Mar 7; 4(5):1423–30.

Toe, Jerry Edidiong Orok and Patrick, Erah (2023). Assessment of knowledge and disposal practices of unused and expired household medicines in a community in Liberia, *Exploratory Research in Clinical and Social Pharmacy,* Volume 12, 2023, 100369, ISSN 2667–2766, https://doi.org/10.1016/j.rcsop.2023.100369.

UK (2013). The National Health Service (Pharmaceutical and Local Pharmaceutical Services) Regulations 2013. http://www.Legislation.gov.uk/uksi/2013/349/pdfs/uksi_20130349_en.pdf.

US Food and Drug Administration. For consumers: how to dispose of unused medicines. Available at: http://www.fda.gov/downloads/Drugs/ResourcesForYou/Consumers/BuyingUsingMedicineSafely/UnderstandingOver-the-Counter Medicines /ucm107163.pdf

USEPA (U.S. Environmental Protection) (2011) Code of federal regulations. Protection of environment: criteria for municipal solid waste landfills. Available at: Http://Www.Gpo.Gov/ Fdsys/Pkg/Cfr-2012-Title40-Vol26/Xml/Cfr-2012-Title40-Vol26-Part258.Xml.

USEPA (United State Environmental Protection Agency) (2010). Landfill recovery and use in Nigeria (Pre-feasibility studies of using Landfill Gas Energy (LFGE)). A report prepared by Centre for People and Environment (CPE).

USFD (2022). Drug Disposal: Drug Take Back Locations| FDA. US Food and Drugs Administration. Available via https://www.fda.gov/drugs/disposal-unused-medicines-what-you-should-know/drug-disposal-drug-take-back-locations (Accessed 11 August 2022).

USFD (2022). Where and How to Dispose of Unused Medicines | FDA. Available via https://www.fda.gov/consumers/consumer-updates/where-and-how-dispose -unused-medicines (Accessed 11 August 2022).

Vatovec, C., van Wagoner, E. and Evans, C. (2017). Investigating sources of pharmaceutical pollution: survey of over-the-counter and prescription medication purchasing, use, and disposal practices among university students. *J Environ Manage,* 198:348–52.

Vellinga, A., Cormican, S., Driscoll, J., Furey, M., O'Sullivan, M. and Cormican, M. (2014). Public practice regarding disposal of unused medicines in Ireland. *Sci Total Environ*, 478:98–102.

Verlicchi, P., Al Aukidy, M., Galletti, A., Petrovic, M. and Barcel, D. (2012). Hospital effluent: Investigation of the concentrations and distribution of pharmaceuticals and environmental risk assessment. Sci Total Environ. 2012; 430:109-18. DOI: 10.1016/j.scitotenv.2012.04.055

Vollmer, G. (2010). Disposal of pharmaceutical waste in households–a European survey. In: Kümmerer K, Hempel M. (eds) *Green and Sustainable pharmacy*. Springer, Berlin, Heidelberg, pp 165–78, 2010.

Wang, X.P. Howley, A.B. Boxall and Rudd, M.A. (2016). Behaviour, preferences, and willingness to pay for measures aimed at preventing pollution by pharmaceuticals and personal care products in China. *Integr Environ Assess Manag,* 12 (4), pp. 793–800, 10.1002/ieam.1746.

West, L.M., Diak, L., Cordina, M. and Stewart, D. (2014). A systematic review of the literature on 'medication wastage': an exploration of causative factors and effects of interventions. *Int J Clin Pharm* 36(5):873–881.

West, L.M. (2015). Medication wastage: the current situation.

Wieczorkiewicz, S.M., Kassamali, Z. and Danziger, L.H. (2013). Behind closed doors: medication storage and disposal in the home. *Ann Pharmacother* 47(4):482–489.

Wondimu, A., Molla, F., Demeke, B., Eticha, T., Assen, A., Abrha, S. and Melkam, W. (2015). Household storage of medicines and associated factors in Tigray Region, Northern Ethiopia. *PloS One*, 10(8):e0135650.

World Health Organization (2019). Guidelines for safe disposal of unwanted pharmaceuticals in and after emergencies. WHO/EDM/PAR/99.2. Department of Essential Drugs and Other Medicines, World Health Organization, Switzerland.

Yanovitzky, I. (2016). The American medicine chest challenge: Evaluation of adrugtake-back and disposal campaign. *J Stud Alcohol Drugs.* 2016; 77(4):549–55. DOI: 10.15288/jsad.2016.77.549

Zuccato, E., Castiglioni, S., Fanelli, R., Bagnati, R., Reitano, G. and Calamari, D. (2004). Risks related to the discharge of pharmaceuticals in the environment: further research is needed. In: Kümmerer K. (eds) *Pharmaceuticals in the Environment.* Springer, Berlin, Heidelberg, pp. 431–7, 2004.

Zuccato, E., Castiglioni, S., Fanelli, R., Reitano, G., Bagnati, R. and Chiabrando, C. (2006). Pharmaceuticals in the environmentinItaly: causes, occurrence, effects and control. *Environ Sci Pollut Res Int.* 2006; 13(1): 15–21. DOI: 10.1065/espr2006.01.004.

Glimpses of Survey Work

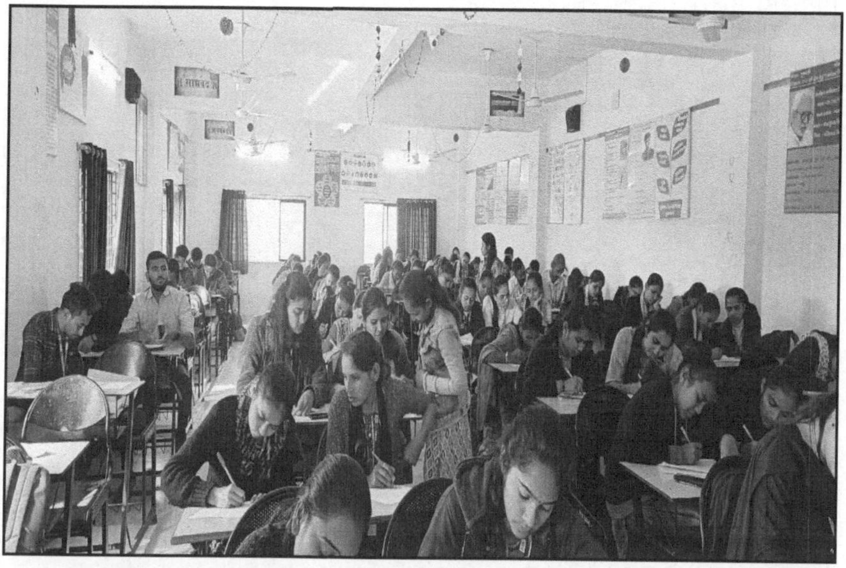

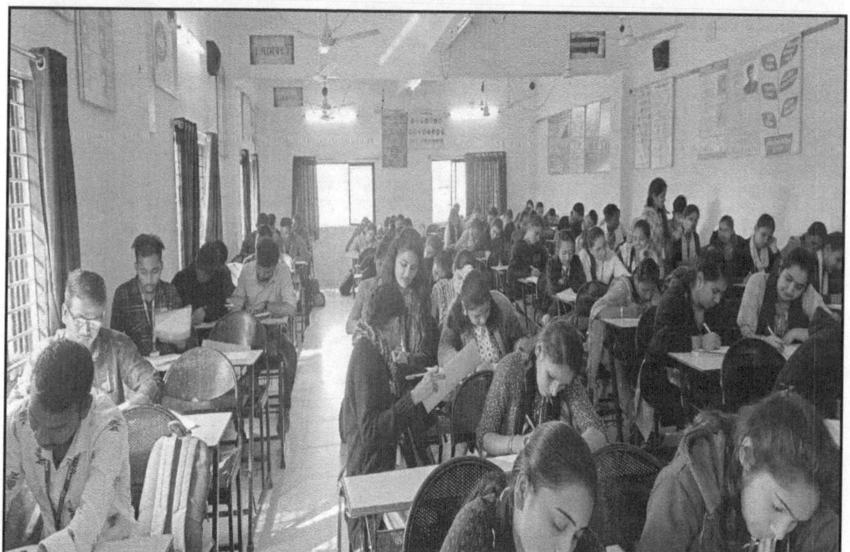

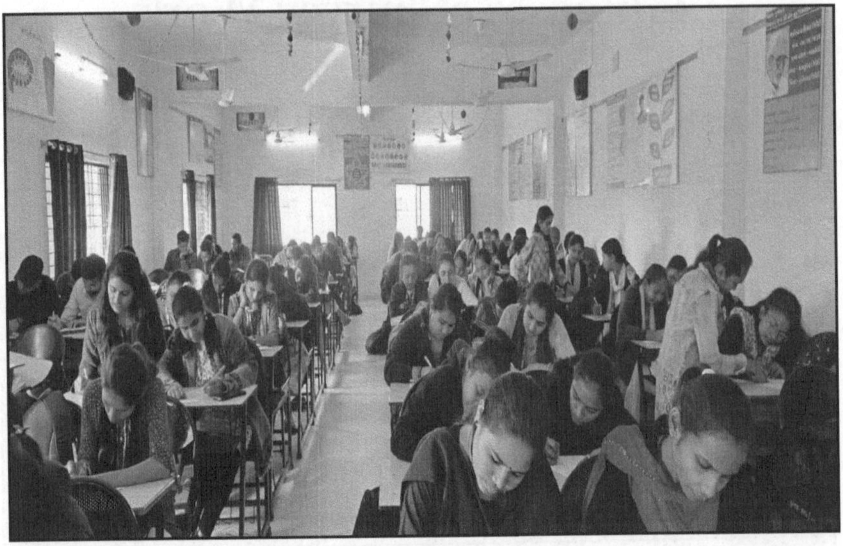

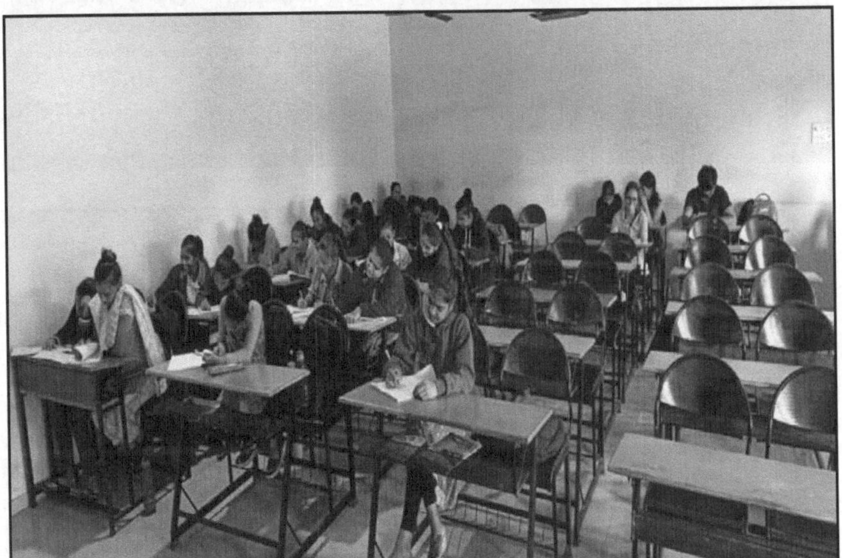

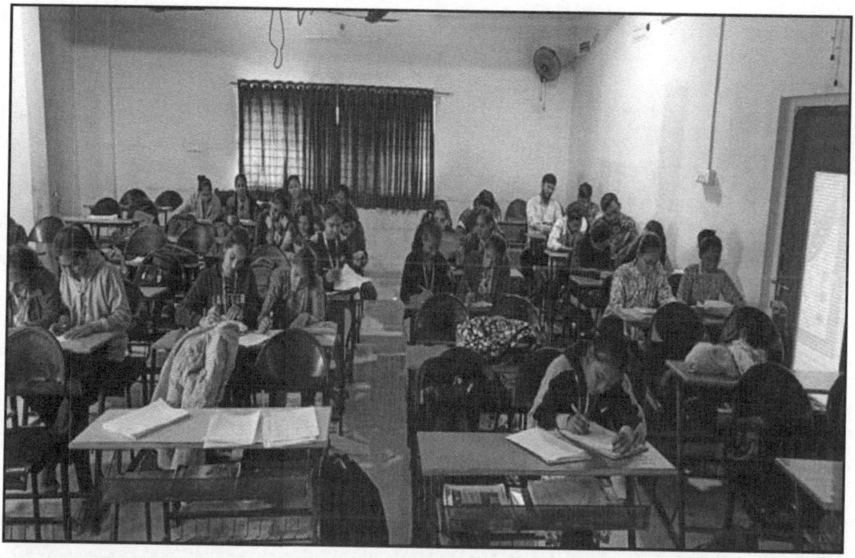

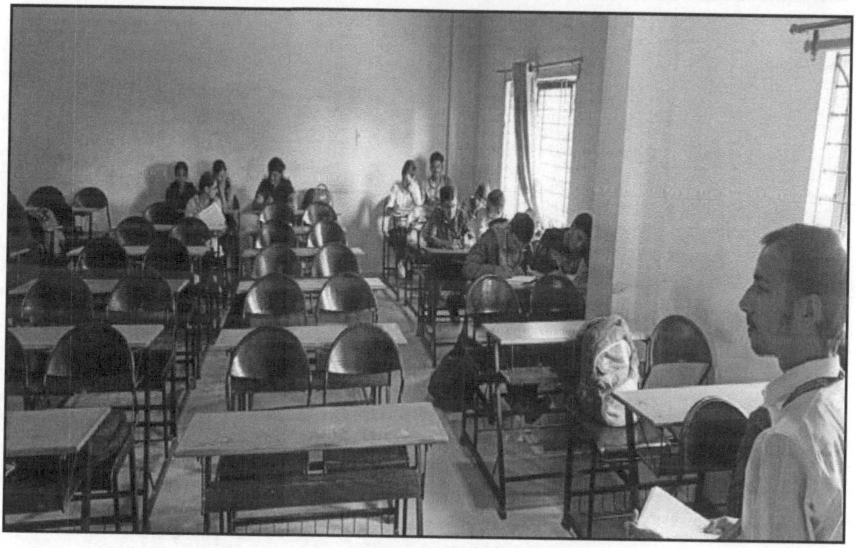

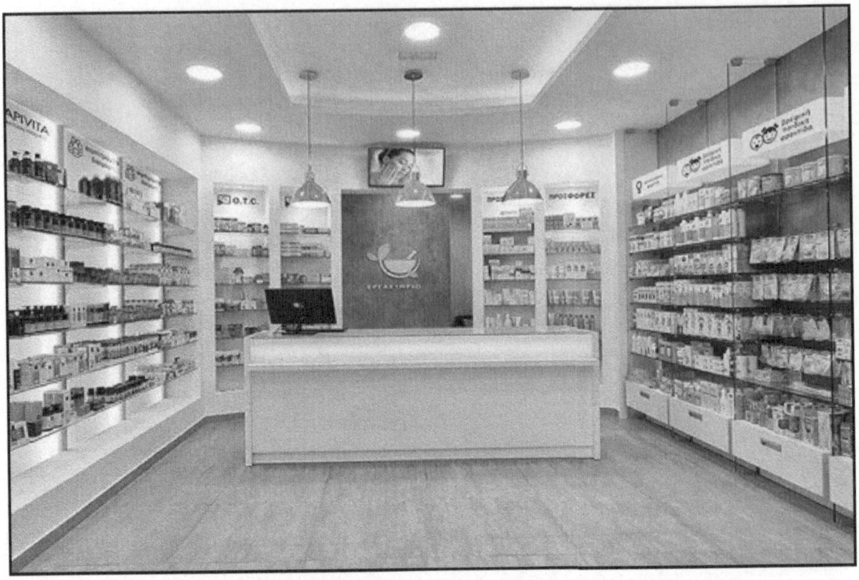
APIVITA
O.T.C.
ΠΡΟΣΦΟΡΕΣ

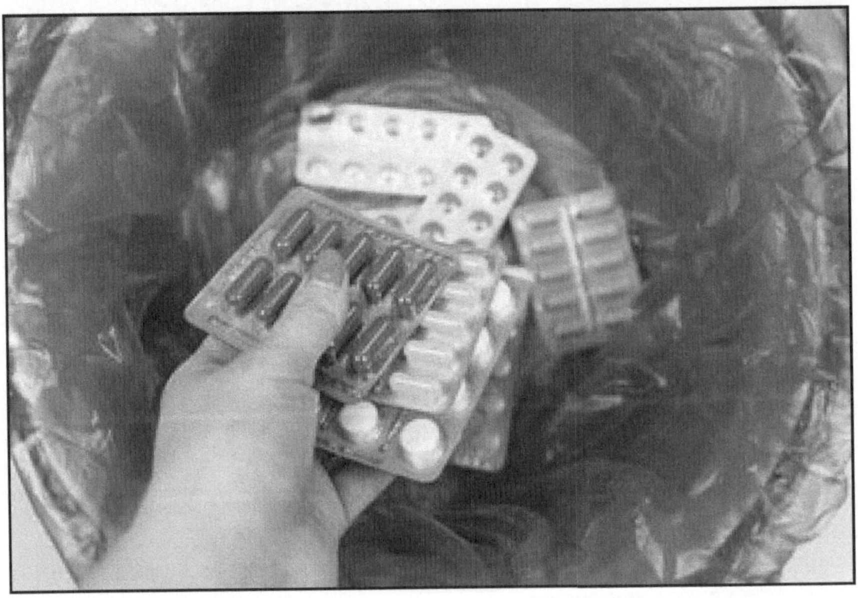

ANNEXURE I

Study of Awareness and Knowledge about Disposal of Unused and Expired Medication among Professional and Students in Gujarat, India.

ગુજરાતમાં વ્યવસાયિકો અને વિદ્યાર્થીઓમાં વણવપરાયેલી

અને સમય અવધિ સમાપ્ત થયેલ

દવાઓના નિકાલ અંગે જાગૃતિ અને જ્ઞાનનો અભ્યાસ

વ્યવસાયિક પ્રશ્નાવલી/વિદ્યાર્થી પ્રશ્નાવલી

[1] *General Information* સામાન્ય માહિતી

<table>
<tr><td>1. Locality (વિસ્તાર)- Village (ગામ)/Semi Urban (અર્ધ-શહેરી)/Urban (શહેર)</td><td colspan="2">2. Location (વિસ્તાર)</td></tr>
<tr><td>3. Taluka/Tehsil (તાલુકા)</td><td colspan="2">4. District (જીલ્લો)</td></tr>
<tr><td colspan="3">5. Respondent (ઉત્તરદાતા) (tick √): 1. Pharmacy Student (ફાર્મસી વિદ્યાર્થી);
2. Nursing student (નર્સિંગ વિદ્યાર્થીઓ); 3. Trainee Teacher student (તાલીમાર્થી શિક્ષકો/વિદ્યાર્થીઓ); 4. College Teachers (કોલેજ શિક્ષકો);
5. Households (ગૃહસ્થ), 6. Others (specify) અન્ય (સ્પષ્ટ કરો)</td></tr>
<tr><td colspan="3">6. Name (ઉત્તરદાતાનું નામ)</td></tr>
<tr><td colspan="2">7. Mobile Number (મોબાઇલ નંબર)</td><td>8. Type of Mobile મોબાઇલનો પ્રકાર-Simple/Android એન્ડ્રોઇડ</td></tr>
<tr><td colspan="2">9. Gender લિંગ (Male પુરુષ/Female સ્ત્રી)</td><td>10. Age ઉંમર (years વર્ષ)</td></tr>
<tr><td colspan="3">11. Occupation (વ્યવસાય/ધંધો) 1. Students (વિદ્યાર્થી);
2. Professional (વ્યાવસાયિક); 3. Service (નોકરી); 4. Labor (મજૂર);
5. Crop Farming (ખેતી); 6. Dairy (પશુપાલન); 7. Farm labor (ખેત મજૂર); 8. Others specify (અન્ય સ્પષ્ટ કરો)</td></tr>
<tr><td>12. Education (years) શિક્ષણ (વર્ષ)</td><td colspan="2">13. સામાજિક જૂથ Social Group- Scheduled Caste અનુસૂચિત જાતિ= 1; Scheduled Tribe અનુસૂચિત જનજાતિ = 2, OBC અન્ય પછાત વર્ગો= 3; General સામાન્ય = 4</td></tr>
</table>

14. Marital status વૈવાહિક સ્થિતિ - Single અપરિણીત, Married પરિણીત, Divorced, છૂટાછેડા લીધેલ, Widowed વિધવા	15. Family type કૌટુંબિક પ્રકાર: Joint સંયુક્ત//Nuclear વિભક્ત:			
16. Family size (No.) કુટુંબનું કદ	Adult Male પુખ્ત પુરૂષ	Adult Female પુખ્ત સ્ત્રી	Children (up to 15 years) M&f બાળકો (15 વર્ષ સુધી- છોકરા-છોકરી)	
17. Experience in Profession (years) વ્યવસાયમાં અનુભવ (વર્ષો)	18. Income group આવક શ્રેણી APL/BPL/AAY:			

[2] *About Use of Medication* દવાના ઉપયોગ વિશે

Sl	*Particulars*	*1*	*2*	*3*	*4*	*5*
1.	Frequency of medications storage at household ઘરેલુ દવાઓના સંગ્રહની પ્રવૃત્તિનું આવર્તન	Always હંમેશા	Often ઘણીવાર	Sometimes ક્યારેક	Rare ભાગ્યે જ	Never ક્યારેય નહીં
2.	Medicine Storage location at home ઘરે દવાનું સંગ્રહ સ્થાન	Loker લોકર	Refrigerator રેફ્રિજરેટર	Bedroom બેડરૂમ	living room લિવિંગ રૂમ	don't know ખબર નથી
3.	If needed, storing of medication away from moisture, light and high temperature (more than 25° C) is practiced in household જો જરૂરી હોય તો, ઘરમાં ભેજ, પ્રકાશ અને ઊંચા તાપમાન (25°સે થી વધુ) થી દૂર દવાનો સંગ્રહ કરવામાં આવે છે/કરો છો.	Always હંમેશા	Often ઘણી વાર	Sometimes ક્યારેક	Rare ભાગ્યે જ	Neverક્યારેય નહીં
4.	Use of any prescribed medication for a relative or a friend કોઈ સંબંધી અથવા મિત્રે સૂચવેલ કોઈપણ દવાનો ઉપયોગ કરવામાં આવે છે	Always હંમેશા	Often ઘણી વાર	Sometimes ક્યારેક	Rare ભાગ્યે જ	Never ક્યારેય નહીં

5.	Do you check the expiration date of the medicine before buying it? શું તમે દવા ખરીદતા પહેલા તેની અવધિ સમાપ્ત તારીખ તપાસો છો?	Always હંમેશા	Often ઘણી વાર	Sometimes ક્યારેક	Rare ભાગ્યે જ	Never ક્યારેય નહીં
6.	Verification of expiry date before administering medications દવાઓ આપતા પહેલા અવધિ સમાપ્ત તારીખની ચકાસણી કરો	Always હંમેશ	Often ઘણી	Sometimes ક્યારે	Rare ભાગ્યે	Never ક્યારેય નહી

[3] About Used and Expired Medication at home ન વપરાયેલી અને સમયસીમા સમાપ્ત થઈ ગયેલી દવાઓ વિશે

1.	Purchased medicines remaining unused at home among household ખરીદેલી દવાઓ ઘરમાં વણવપરાયેલ પડી રહી છે	Yes/No- હા/ના				
2.	If yes, type of medication remaining unused at home among household જો હા, તો ઘરમાં વણવપરાયેલ દવાઓનો પ્રકાર (tick √)	Tablets ટેબ્લેટ	Capsule કેપ્સ્યુલ	Liquid/Syrup લિક્વિડ સીરપ	Powder પાવડર	Other અન્ય
	A. Analgesic (pain killer) પીડાનાશક (પેઇન કિલર)					
	B. Antibiotic (destroying bacteria and curing infections) એન્ટિબાયોટિક (બેક્ટેરિયાનો નાશ કરે છે અને ચેપ મટાડે છે)					
	C. Antihypertensive (for hypertension) એન્ટિહાઇપરટેન્સિવ (હાયપરટેન્શન માટે)					
	D. Antidiabetic (blood glucose control) એન્ટિડાયાબિટીક (બ્લડ ગ્લુકોઝ નિયંત્રણ)					
	E. Digestion (for digest and constipation) પાચન (પાચન અને કબજિયાત માટે)					

	F. Skin disease (dermatology) ત્વચા રોગ (ત્વચારોગવિજ્ઞાન)					
	G. Other medication અન્ય દવા					
3.	Number of unused medications stored in household ઘરમાં સંગ્રહિત વણવપરાયેલ દવાઓની સંખ્યા	0-5	6-10	11-15	16-20	More than 20
4.	Classes of unused medications that are in your household તમારા ઘરમાં વણવપરાયેલ દવાઓના વર્ગો (tick √)	Prescribed medication નિયત દવા	Non-prescribed medication બિન-નિર્ધારિત દવા	Sub-cutaneous injection સબક્યુટેનીયસ ઈન્જેક્શન	Intr-avenous injection નસમાં ઇન્જેક્શન	Patches પેચો
5.	Number of expired medication stored in household ઘરમાં તારીખ અવધિ સમાપ્ત થયેલ દવાઓની સંખ્યા (tick √)	0-5	6-10	11-15	16-20	More than 20
6.	Classes of expired medications that are in your household દવાની તારીખ અવધિ સમાપ્ત થયેલ દવાઓના પ્રકારો કે જે તમારા ઘરમાં છે (tick √)	Prescribed medication નિયત દવા	Non-prescribed medication બિનનિર્ધારિત દવા	Subcutaneous injection સબક્યુટેનીયસ ઈન્જેક્શન	Intr-avenous injection નસમાં ઇન્જેક્શન	Patches પેચો

[4] Reasons for Keeping Purchased Medicine unused at home ખરીદેલ દવાને ઘરે ન વપરાયેલ રાખવાના કારણો

Sl.	*Reasons for Possessing Unused Medication*	*(tick √)*
1.	Disease or condition resolve/symptoms improved રોગ અથવા સ્થિતિનું નિરાકરણ/રોગનું નિરાકરણ/આરોગ્યમાં સુધારો	
2.	Forgetting to take medicine દવા લેવાનું ભૂલી ગયા	
3.	Change of medication by the doctor ડૉક્ટર દ્વારા દવામાં ફેરફાર	
4.	Experiencing side-effect આડઅસરનો અનુભવ થાય	
5.	Taste is bitter સ્વાદ કડવો છે	
6.	Busy schedule વ્યસ્ત સમયપત્રક	
7.	Change of doctor/Change to another treatment ડૉક્ટરની બદલી/અન્ય સારવારમાં બદલાવ	

Sl.	*Reasons for Possessing Unused Medication*	*(tick √)*
8.	Excess quantity supplied વધારાનો જથ્થો પૂરો પાડવામાં આવ્યો	
9.	Inconvenience/Difficulty following instructions સૂચનાઓનું પાલન કરવામાં અસુવિધા/મુશ્કેલી	
10.	Medicine label had unclear instruction દવાના લેબલમાં અસ્પષ્ટ સૂચના હતી	
11.	Other અન્ય	

[5] Knowledge on Disposal of Unused and Expired Medication ન વપરાયેલ અને સમયસીમા સમાપ્ત થયેલ દવાઓના નિકાલ અંગેની જાણકારી

No.	*Questions*	*Yes* હા/ નાં*No*
A.	**Unused** વણવપરાયેલ દવા	
1.	Do you know that misused/repeated change or not complete antibiotics may cause drug resistance? શું તમે જાણો છો કે દુરુપયોગ/પુનરાવર્તિત ફેરફાર અથવા સંપૂર્ણ એન્ટિબાયોટિક્સ ડ્રગ પ્રતિકારનું કારણ બની શકે છે?	
2.	Do you know about "drug-take-back system"? શું તમે "ડ્રગ-ટેક-બેક સિસ્ટમ" વિશે જાણો છો?	
3.	Do you separate unused medicine before disposal? Yes/No શું તમે ન વપરાયેલ દવાને નિકાલ કરતા પહેલા અલગ કરો છો? હા નાં	
B.	**Expired** સમય અવધિ સમાપ્ત થયેલ દવાઓ	
1.	Do you know about medication waste? શું તમે દવાના કચરા વિશે જાણો છો?	
2.	Have you ever read medicines disposal instruction? શું તમે ક્યારેય દવાઓના નિકાલ માટેની સૂચનાઓ વાંચી છે?	
3.	Have you ever followed medicines disposal instruction? શું તમે ક્યારેય દવાઓના નિકાલ માટેની સૂચનાઓનું પાલન કર્યું છે?	
4.	Do you know that improper disposal of unused and expired medicines can affect the environment and health? શું તમે જાણો છો કે	

No.	*Questions*	*Yes* હા/ ના*No*
	બિનઉપયોગી અને સમયસીમા સમાપ્ત થયેલ દવાઓનો અયોગ્ય નિકાલ પર્યાવરણ અને આરોગ્યને અસર કરી શકે છે?	
5.	Have you Received education regarding safe disposal of medication? Yes/No શું તમે દવાના સુરક્ષિત નિકાલ અંગેનું શિક્ષણ મેળવ્યું છે? હા નાં	
6.	How often you seek information from official resources safe disposals of medications (Always, Often, Sometimes, Rare, Never) શું તમે દવાના સુરક્ષિત નિકાલ અંગેનું શિક્ષણ મેળવ્યું છે?	

[6] Actions to minimize or control the hazardous effect of unused and expired medicines ન વપરાયેલ અને સમયસીમા સમાપ્ત થયેલ દવાઓની જોખમી અસરને ઘટાડવા અથવા નિયંત્રિત કરવા માટેની ક્રિયાઓ

Sl.	*Details*	*(tick √)*
1.	By providing proper guidance to the consumer ગ્રાહકને યોગ્ય માર્ગદર્શન આપીને	
2.	By prescribing in quantities and for duration that ensure patient compliance જથ્થામાં અને સમયગાળા માટે સૂચવીને જે દર્દીના પાલનની ખાતરી કરે છે	
3.	By donating the unused medicines વણવપરાયેલ દવા દવાઓનું દાન કરીને	
4.	By depositing unused medicine in nearby Public Health Centre બિનઉપયોગી દવા નજીકના જાહેર આરોગ્ય કેન્દ્રમાં જમા કરાવીને	
5.	By consuming the same as per doctor advice ડૉક્ટરની સલાહ મુજબ જ સેવન કરવું	
6.	Lowering the number of prescribed medicines by doctor ડૉક્ટર દ્વારા સૂચવવામાં આવેલી દવાઓની સંખ્યા ઘટાડવી	
7.	Other અન્ય	

[7] Disposal practice of unused medicines among households ઘરોમાં ન વપરાયેલ દવાઓના નિકાલની રીત/કેવી રીતે કરશો?

Sl.	*Disposal Practice of Unused Medicines*	*(tick √)*
1.	Throwing them away in household garbage તેમને ઘરના કચરામાં ફેંકી દેવા	
2.	Donating them to hospital તેમને હૉસ્પિટલ માટે દાન	
3.	Giving them to friends or relatives તેમને મિત્રો અથવા સંબંધીઓને આપવું	
4.	Returning them back to pharmacy તેમને ફાર્મસીમાં પાછા ફર્યા	
5.	Returning to Hospital હૉસ્પિટલમાં પરત ફર્યા	
6.	Keeping them at home until expired સમાપ્ત થાય ત્યાં સુધી તેમને ઘરે રાખવા	
7.	Flushing them in toilet તેમને શૌચાલયમાં ફ્લશ કરવું	
8.	Burning them તેને બાળી દો	
9.	Lowering the number of prescribed medicines by doctors ડોકટરો દ્વારા સૂચવવામાં આવેલી દવાઓની સંખ્યા ઘટાડવી	
10.	Give/donate medication to other people અન્ય લોકોને દવા આપો/દાન કરો	
11.	I do not dispose medication હું દવાનો નિકાલ કરતો નથી	

[8] Disposal practice of expired medicines among households ઘરોમાં સમયસીમા સમાપ્ત થયેલ દવાઓના નિકાલની રીત

Sl.	*Disposal Practice of Expired Medicines*	*(tick √)*
1.	Throwing them away in household garbage તેમને ઘરના કચરામાં ફેંકી દેવા	
2.	Flushing them in toilet તેમને શૌચાલયમાં ફ્લશ કરવું	
3.	Burning them તેને બાળી દો	
4.	I do not dispose medication હું દવાનો નિકાલ કરતો નથી	
5.	Do not know ખબર નથી	

[9] Bodies responsible for Creation of Awareness about Disposal of Unused and Expired Medication ન વપરાયેલઅને સમયસીમા સમાપ્ત થયેલ દવાઓના નિકાલ અંગે જાગૃતિના નિર્માણ માટે જવાબદાર સંસ્થાઓ

Sl.	*Bodies*	*(tick √)*
1.	Physician/Doctor ફિઝિશિયન/ડૉક્ટર	
2.	Pharmacist/Chemist shop ફાર્માસિસ્ટ/કેમિસ્ટની દુકાન	
3.	Pharmaceutical industries ફાર્માસ્યુટિકલ ઉદ્યોગો	
4.	Every health professional દરેક આરોગ્ય વ્યાવસાયિક	
5.	Government સરકાર	
6.	NGOs એનજીઓ	
7.	Health bureau આરોગ્ય બ્યુરો	
8.	Environment agency પર્યાવરણ એજન્સી	
9.	Drug regulatory agency ડ્રગ રેગ્યુલેટરી એજન્સી	
10.	Others અન્ય	

[10] Best/Preferred method for Creation of Awareness about Disposal of Unused and Expired Medication ન વપરાયેલ અને સમયસીમા સમાપ્ત થયેલ દવાઓના નિકાલ અંગે જાગૃતિ ઉભી કરવા માટેની શ્રેષ્ઠ/પસંદગીની પદ્ધતિ

Sl.	*Bodies*	*Tick (multiple responses)*
1.	Awareness program in every village/hospital દરેક ગામ/હોસ્પિટલમાં જાગૃતિ કાર્યક્રમ દ્વારા	
2.	Hoardings/Posters/Pamplets હોર્ડિંગ્સ/પોસ્ટર્સ/પેમ્પલેટ્સ દ્વારા	
3.	Newspaper/Magazines અખબાર/મેગેઝિન દ્વારા	
4.	Air and Electronic media (Program on TV, Radio) એર અને ઇલેક્ટ્રોનિક મીડિયા (ટીવી, રેડિયો પર પ્રોગ્રામ) દ્વારા	

5.	Digital Media (Youtube, Facebook, Whatsup, instagram) ડિજિટલ મીડિયા (યુટ્યુબ, ફેસબુક, વોટ્સઅપ, ઇન્સ્ટાગ્રામ)	
6.	Introducing the topic on School Curriculum શાળાના અભ્યાસક્રમ પર વિષયનો પરિચય દ્વારા	
7.	Mobile dialer tone like Covid19 કોવિડ19 જેવો મોબાઈલ ડાયલર ટોન દ્વારા	
8.	Text messages on Mobile મોબાઇલ પર ટેક્સ્ટ સંદેશાઓ દ્વારા	
9.	Others અન્ય	

[11] Perceptions towards Disposal of Unused/Expired Medicines ન વપરાયેલ અને સમયસીમા સમાપ્ત થયેલ દવાઓના નિકાલ પ્રત્યેની ધારણા (tick √)

Sr. No.	*Statement* નિવેદન	*Strongly Agree* જોરદાર રીતેસંમત	*Slightly Agree* સહેજ સંમત	*Agree* સંમત	*Disagree* અસંમત	*Strongly Disagree* ભારપૂર્વકઅ સંમત
1.	Unused medicines should not be thrown into dustbins ન વપરાયેલ દવાઓ કચરાપેટીમાં ફેંકવી જોઈએ નહીં					
2.	Burning of expired medicines can release toxic substances which can be inhaledby the people સમયસીમા સમાપ્ત થયેલ દવાઓને બાળવાથી ઝેરી પદાર્થો બહાર નીકળી શકે છે જે લોકો શ્વાસમાં લઈ શકે છે					
3.	Unsafe practices of medicines disposal can pollute the environment દવાઓના નિકાલની અસુરક્ષિત પદ્ધતિઓ પર્યાવરણને પ્રદૂષિત કરી શકે છે					

Sr. No.	*Statement* નિવેદન	*Strongly Agree* જોરદાર રીતેસંમત	*Slightly Agree* સહેજ સંમત	*Agree* સંમત	*Disagree* અસંમત	*Strongly Disagree* ભારપૂર્વકઅ સંમત
4.	There should be a public awareness program about the harmful effects ofimproper medicine disposal practices દવાના નિકાલની અયોગ્ય પદ્ધતિઓના નુકસાનકારક અસરો વિશે જનજાગૃતિ કાર્યક્રમ હોવો જોઈએ					
5.	Community pharmacists have an important role in mitigating the problem ofimproper medicine disposal practices સામુદાયિક ફાર્માસિસ્ટની દવાના નિકાલની અયોગ્ય પ્રેક્ટિસની સમસ્યાને ઘટાડવામાં મહત્વની ભૂમિકા હોય છે.					
6.	Unused and expired medicines present potential risks at home ન વપરાયેલ અને સમયસીમા સમાપ્ત થયેલ દવાઓ ઘર પર સંભવિત જોખમો રજૂ કરે છે					
7.	There is a lack of adequate information on the safe disposal of unused medicines ન વપરાયેલ દવાઓના સુરક્ષિત નિકાલ અંગે પૂરતી માહિતીનો અભાવ છે					
8.	Children are more vulnerable to the risks associated with unused and expiredhousehold medicines બાળકો ન વપરાયેલ અને સમાપ્ત થયેલ ઘરગથ્થુ દવાઓ સાથે સંકળાયેલા જોખમો માટે વધુ સંવેદનશીલ હોય છે					

Sr. No.	*Statement* નિવેદન	*Strongly Agree* જોરદાર રીતેસંમત	*Slightly Agree* સહેજ સંમત	*Agree* સંમત	*Disagree* અસંમત	*Strongly Disagree* ભારપૂર્વકઅ સંમત
9.	Doctors and health professionals should provide advice on the safe disposal ofunused and expired household medicines ડોકટરો અને આરોગ્ય વ્યવસાયિકોએ ન વપરાયેલ અને સમયસીમા સમાપ્ત થયેલ ગયેલી ઘરગથ્થુ દવાઓના સુરક્ષિત નિકાલ અંગે સલાહ આપવી જોઈએ					
10.	Drug take-back programs for unused and expired medicines should bemandatory ન વપરાયેલ અને સમયસીમા સમાપ્ત થયેલ દવાઓ માટે ડ્રગ ટેક-બેક પ્રોગ્રામ ફરજિયાત હોવા જોઈએ					
11	Outreach and awareness programs about how to dispose of unused and expiredmedicines should be initiated ન વપરાયેલ અને સમયસીમા સમાપ્ત થયેલ દવાઓનો નિકાલ કેવી રીતે કરવો તે અંગે આઉટરીચ અને જાગૃતિ કાર્યક્રમો શરૂ કરવા જોઈએ.					

[12] Suggestions

1.	Do you think that there is a need for a program to collect unused medicines from home? શું તમને લાગે છે કે ઘરેથી ન વપરાયેલ દવાઓ એકત્રિત કરવા માટે કોઈ પ્રોગ્રામની જરૂર છે?	Yes/No
2.	Do you think that consumers should be made more aware about the hazards of unsafe disposal & methods of safe disposal? શું તમને લાગે છે કે ગ્રાહકોને અસુરક્ષિત નિકાલના જોખમો અને સલામત નિકાલની પદ્ધતિઓ વિશે વધુ જાગૃત કરવા જોઈએ?	Yes/No
3.	What measures do you suggest to improve awareness of consumers regarding safe disposal of medicines? દવાઓના સુરક્ષિત નિકાલ અંગે ગ્રાહકોની જાગૃતિ વધારવા માટે તમે કયા પગલાં સૂચવો છો?	
	1.	
	2.	
	3.	

ANNEXURE II

Study of Awareness and Knowledge about Disposal of Unused and Expired Medication among Professional and Students in Gujarat, India

The pharmacies are requested to provide the information related to disposal of unused and expired medicines in your pharmacy. This information will be strictly used for research purpose only.

1.	Name of Pharmacist	
2.	Locality (Village/Semi Urban/Urban)	
3.	Place of Pharmacy	
4.	Taluka/Tehsil	Anand
5.	District	Anand
6.	About Registration	Registered Pharmacists/Unregistered
7.	Education level	
8.	Gender (male/Female)	
9.	Age (years)	
10.	Experience of Pharmacy (years)	
11.	Do you (pharmacies) ensure proper storage and segregation of date expired drugs?	Yes/No
12.	What are the current procedures for identifying expired medications in your pharmacy?	(a) Regular checks of medication (b) Alerts from computer software (c) Brought to notice by Consumer (d) Any other

13.	What are the current procedures for managing expired medications in your pharmacy?	(a) Separation of expired medicines and Return to Pharmaceutical distributor (b) Separation of expired medicines and proper disposal of expired medicines (c) Incinerate through drug inspectorate (d) Dispose pf workplace garbage
14.	Should drug distributors or whole- salers collect back their date expired drugs?	Yes/No
15.	Have you dispose of expired drugs safely, without harming people or the environment (as per stipulated guidelines)	Yes/No
16.	Do you educate customers about the proper disposal of expired medicines?	Yes/No
17.	Do you have policy to take back unused drugs from consumers?	Yes/No
18.	If yes, How many consumers generally return unused drugs in a month? (out of 100, how many return)	
19.	Does consumer check the expiry date on medicine while purchasing/taking to home?	Yes/No
20.	If yes, how many consumers generally check expiry date while taking medicine to home? (out of 100, how many return)	
21a.	How many consumers buy medicine as per prescription (out of 100, how many)	

21b.	How many consumers buy medicine as per their own knowledge (out of 100, how many)	
21c.	How many consumers buy medicine as per your advice (out of 100, how many)	
22.	How many consumers ask you about procedure to dispose off date expired medicines? (out of 100, how many)	
23.	Do you provide information about proper medication disposal practices to patients?	Yes/No
24.	What are the biggest challenges you face in safely disposing of expired medications?	(a) Lack of standard protocols (b) Improper disposal practices (c) Environmental concerns (d) Lack of trained personal (e) Financial constraints
25.	What changes or improvements would you suggest to enhance the safe disposal of expired medicines?	(a) Massive awareness programs for consumers (b) Collection of unused medicines by some NGOs for further used (c) Creating the disposable unit at PHC level
26.	Is there a need for creating the awareness among consumers about drug disposal policy in India?	Yes/No
27.	What are your recommendations for proper disposal of unused and date expired medicine?	(a) Educate patients on how to dispose of medications safely (b) Create standard protocols for disposing of expired medications (c) Create legislation to monitor and control the disposal of unused and expired medications (d) Create programs to collect unwanted drugs from pharmacies

ANNEXURE III

Guidelines for Safe Disposal of Unwanted Pharmaceuticals in and after Emergencies

World Health Organization
Churches' Action for Health of the World Council of Churches ECHO
International Health Services Ltd.
International Committee of the Red Cross
International Federation of Red Cross and Red Crescent Societies
International Pharmaceutical Federation
International Solid Waste Association Médecins Sans Frontières
Office of the United Nations High Commissioner for Refugees OXFAM
Pharmaciens Sans Frontières United Nations Children's Fund
United Nations Industrial Development Organization

1. Introduction

1.1 *Background*

During conflicts and natural disasters large quantities of pharmaceuticals are often donated as part of humanitarian assistance. Undoubtedly many of the pharmaceuticals save lives and alleviate suffering, but some donations given by well-meaning but uninformed people may cause problems. Pharmaceuticals may arrive past or near their expiry date, may be inappropriate for the needs, be unrecognizable because they are labelled in a foreign language or may have been sent in unwanted quantities. Donated pharmaceuticals with a long shelf-life may be mismanaged, particularly in the confusion during and after armed conflict or a natural disaster. Staff and storage space may be lacking and the pharmaceutical management system in disarray. Such problems also occur when drug donations form part of development assistance. Smaller quantities of pharmaceutical waste may accumulate in the absence of emergency situations, due to inadequacies in stock management and distribution, and to lack of a routine system of disposal. Safe disposal of these unwanted or expired drugs often creates a major problem.

These disposal guidelines are based on a report on the safe disposal of unwanted and unusable drugs in Mostar, which had accumulated during the war in Bosnia and Herzegovina. Quantifying pharmacy-eutical waste may be difficult. One report states that 50–60% of the 27, 800–34,800 metric tons of medical supplies donated to Bosnia and Herzegovina between 1992 and mid-1996 were considered to be inappropriate, and by mid-1996 there were an estimated 17,000 metric tons of unusable drugs stockpiled in warehouses and clinics throughout the country. These dramatic figures are contested: something in the region of 1,000 metric tons is considered by some to be more reasonable. A recent figure of 2,000 metric tons of pharmaceutical waste in Croatia is regarded as accurate. Unusable donated drugs hindered the efficient operation of pharmacies in many of the states of the former Yugoslavia and represented a significant disposal problem.

1.2 *Prevention of Waste from Pharmaceutical Donations Appropriate Donations*

Inappropriate donations may be minimized by donors adhering to the interagency *Guidelines for Drug Donations.* The key principles are that drugs donated shall address the expressed needs of the recipients and that the date of expiration on arrival shall be no less than one year, unless there is clear evidence from the recipients that they have the logistic and managerial capacity to store and distribute shorter–dated drugs efficiently. The blind donation of pharmaceuticals based on unsubstantiated assumptions of recipient needs and logistic capacities is a major factor in the production of pharmaceutical waste.

Good Donations May be Wasted

Mismanagement of received donations may turn a good donation into pharmaceutical waste.

1.3 *The Cost of Disposal of Waste Pharmaceuticals*

The Cost of Waste Pharmaceutical High Temperature Incineration

Pharmaceuticals are ideally disposed of by high temperature (i.e. above 1,200°C) incineration. Such incineration facilities, equipped with adequate emission control, are mainly to be found in the industrialized world. Quotations for disposing of the pharmaceutical waste in Croatia and Bosnia and Herzegovina in this way range from US$ 2.2/kg to US$ 4.1/kg. To incinerate the current stockpile of waste pharmaceuticals in Croatia would therefore cost between US$4.4 million and US$ 8.2 million.

Quoted Weights of Pharmaceutical Waste

The gross weights mentioned previously include packaging. Actual pharmaceutical contents may be half, or less than half, of the gross weight.

1.4 *Purpose of the Guidelines*

These guidelines provide advice on the implementation of safe disposal of unusable pharmaceuticals in emergencies and in countries in transition where official assistance and advice may not be available. They are not meant to supersede local, regional or national laws regarding disposal of drugs, but to provide assistance where there is insufficient guidance or none at all.

A number of methods for safe disposal of pharmaceuticals are described. These are methods which involve minimal risks to public health and the environment, and include those suitable for countries with limited resources and equipment. The adoption of the guidelines by ministries of health, environment and other relevant ministries, and their practical application, will contribute to the safe and economical elimination of stockpiles of unusable pharmaceuticals.

The best environmental option for pharmaceutical destruction is purpose-built high temperature incineration with adequate flue gas cleaning. However, this is not the only method that can be used to achieve adequate disposal. Indeed many countries do not possess such a facility. It is for this reason that these guidelines are suggested as practical interim alternatives to assist those charged with the safe disposal of unwanted pharmaceuticals. The current guidelines propose a number of marginally less safe treatments and disposal methods, which are however acceptable from the relative risk point of view, when balanced against the risks related to improper or non-disposal (see Section 1.8).

What the Guidelines do Not Cover

There is no attempt to cover the management of other wastes generated by health institutions, for example, infectious waste, photographic chemicals, solvents, wastes with a high content of heavy metals (e.g. mercury and cadmium), chemical laboratory wastes, or radioactive waste. The management of health care wastes generated in normal conditions (i.e. neither during nor after emergencies) is not included. Specialized advice for these categories of waste is available from WHO.

The wider subject of normal drug supply and management is not covered. This includes drug waste minimization and waste separation within the health institution. It is assumed that management procedures and staffing are in place to cover these aspects. In the event of insufficient qualified staff and management capacity to undertake safe disposal then the pharmaceutical waste must be securely stored.

1.5 *Who will Find the Guidelines Useful?*

These guidelines can be used by all relevant health authorities, competent to authorize the use or disposal of drugs. In many countries drug disposal will also involve environmental and waste management authorities, and experts at ministerial, regional and local level. Depending on the situation in the country, the appropriate authority may be a department responsible for pharmaceutical management within the ministry of health, the drug regulatory authority (if different from the former), a regional or local health authority (pharmaceutical officer) or the ministry of environment, etc. It is the responsibility of the qualified appropriate authority to implement the guidelines in coordination with regional and local health authorities, as well as with the directors of health facilities that face the problems of drug disposal.

A local task force or advisory committee should be established at an early stage to assess, analyse and address the problem of drug disposal, and to monitor activities. Furthermore, it is suggested that such a task force has a maximum of five members and that meetings are held as near to the site of the stockpile as possible. Members may be chosen from:

- the drug regulatory authority or ministry of health;
- the ministry of the environment;
- the audit section of the ministry of health;

- institutional pharmacists;
- a qualified hazardous waste expert may be appointed by the authority to be responsible for pharmaceutical waste disposal. If this is done the person appointed should become a member of the task force. The individual can be an expert in environmental management, a registered water chemist, hydrogeologist or sanitary engineer. The choice of expert depends on the technical problems to be faced.

Nongovernmental organizations with pharmaceutical programmes may also have to deal with unusable waste stocks of pharmaceuticals that require disposal. Disposal should be undertaken in conjunction with the relevant authority where such exists.

In non-emergency situations large stockpiles do not usually accumulate, and waste pharmaceuticals are best disposed of on a routine basis, small quantities at a time. This should be organized on a local and institutional level.

1.6 *Administrative Aspects of Writing–Off Unwanted Pharmaceuticals*

Few countries have adequate administrative provisions for writing–off pharmaceutical stock. In the public sector drugs are the property of the state, for which strict accounting procedures are necessary. If procedures exist at all, they tend to be complicated and time-consuming, and in practice the disposal of expired stock is difficult. This applies both to drugs that are procured through the normal channels and to donated drugs.

Administrative and regulatory procedures concerning safe disposal of pharmaceuticals, that are in line with national drug and environment legislation, should be adopted and implemented in countries that receive drug donations.

Simplifying procedures in general would probably be the best solution. One approach would be to state that donated drugs are not entered into the government inventory or considered state property unless specifically accepted as such. In this case any drug that is not officially accepted can be destroyed without the need for governmental approval; however, correct disposal procedures must be followed. A further solution would be to establish special, simplified, administrative procedures for writing–off unwanted donations.

1.7 *Steps to be Taken*

A series of steps need to be taken when disposing of unwanted pharmaceuticals, and these are briefly summarized below.

Decision

The hospital, district or regional pharmacist or organizations with pharmaceutical programmes decide when action needs to be initiated, because of an accumulation of unwanted pharmaceuticals which are unfit for human consumption and for veterinary treatment.

Approval

Approval and sanctioning of disposal of pharmaceuticals must be sought from the appropriate authority. This authority will differ from country to country and may be the department responsible for pharmaceutical management within the ministry of health, the drug regulatory authority, or the regional or local health authority (pharmaceutical officer). In some countries the ministry of the environment should be involved. The guidelines are particularly useful in emergency situations or for countries in transition where official regulations have not yet been developed. In non-emergency situations when significant quantities of donated pharmaceuticals are disposed of, for whatever reason, it may be necessary and judicious to inform the donor.

Planning

Planning, in terms of funding, necessary expertise, human resources, professional time, space, equipment, material and available disposal options will be required. This is essential before practical steps can be taken to start disposal. To obtain a rough estimate of the volume of materials to be sorted, it is recommended that measurements are made using a tape measure, and conversion from volume of material to weight is made using a density figure of 0.2 metric tons/cubic metre.

Forming Work Teams

Work should be conducted by teams consisting of supervising pharmacists and general medical workers, who are preferably pharmaceutical technicians or experienced pharmaceutical warehouse personnel. The size of each team, and the ratio of experts to workers, will be determined by the volume and composition of the stockpiles, and working conditions at the sites.

Health and Safety of Work Teams

All workers should wear appropriate protective equipment including overalls and boots at all times, and gloves, masks and caps when appropriate. Masks should be worn when tablets or capsules are being crushed as part of the disposal technique (for example, inertization, see Section 2.4) and when there is a risk of powders being liberated. Particular care is required when handling antineoplastics.

Sorting

The objective of sorting is to separate the pharmaceuticals into separate categories for which different disposal methods are required. The separation should be made into those that can be safely used and returned to the pharmaceutical supply system and those that require disposal by different methods. For example, controlled drugs (e.g. narcotics), antineoplastic drugs and antibiotics all require special methods of disposal. Substantial investment in human resources may be required for identifying and separating pharmaceuticals.

Disposal

Disposal options vary considerably between situations, and the ideal solution may not be feasible. The aim of these guidelines is to propose the simplest, safest and most practical alternatives.

Security

Controlled substances (e.g. narcotics and psychotropics) require tight security and control. In some countries, scavenging of material from landfills is a frequent problem, and, disposed drugs may be recovered and sold by the scavengers.

Measures are therefore necessary to prevent diversion during sorting, and pilfering of drugs from landfills. Immobilization (see Sections 2.3 and 2.4) is the best method of preventing pilfering from a store or landfill. If, as a last resort, pharmaceuticals must be discarded direct to a landfill then they must be covered immediately with a large quantity of municipal waste.

1.8 *Consequences of Improper Disposal or Non-Disposal*

In general, expired pharmaceuticals do not represent a serious threat to public health or to the environment. Improper disposal may be hazardous if it leads to contamination of water supplies or local sources used by nearby communities or wildlife. Expired drugs may come into the hands of scavengers and children if a landfill is insecure. Pilfering from a stockpile of waste drugs or during sorting may result in expired drugs being diverted to the market for resale and misuse. Most pharmaceuticals past their expiry date become less efficacious and a few may develop a different adverse drug reaction profile. There are some categories of expired drugs or defective disposal practices that carry a public health risk. The main health risks are summarized below.

- Contamination of drinking water must be avoided. Landfills must be sited and constructed in a way that minimizes the possibility of leachate entering an aquifer, surface water or drinking water system.
- Non-biodegradable antibiotics, antineoplastics and disinfectants should not be disposed of into the sewage system as they may kill bacteria necessary for the treatment of sewage. Antineoplastics should not be flushed into watercourses as they may damage aquatic life or contaminate drinking water. Similarly, large quantities of disinfectants should not be discharged into a sewerage system or watercourse but can be introduced if well diluted.
- Burning pharmaceuticals at low temperatures or in open containers results in release of toxic pollutants into the air. Ideally this should be avoided.
- Inefficient and insecure sorting and disposal may allow drugs beyond their expiry date to be diverted for resale to the general public. In some countries scavenging in unprotected insecure landfills is a hazard.
- In the absence of suitable disposal sites and qualified personnel to supervise disposal, unwanted pharmaceuticals present no risk provided they are securely stored in dry conditions. If stored in their original packing there is a risk of diversion and to avoid this they are best stored in drums with the pharmaceuticals immobilized, as described in Section 2.3 on waste encapsulation.

1.9 *Public Information*

The public should be informed about the problem of safe disposal of donated expired pharmaceuticals. Key points to present to the media are:

1. the vast majority of pharmaceuticals are donated with the intention to help; there are only rare occurrences of "dumping" by unscrupulous companies to gain tax relief or off-load unwanted stock;
2. when pharmaceuticals pass their expiry date they do not automatically become hazardous, they simply becomes less efficacious;
3. most pharmaceuticals are relatively harmless to the environment; they do not present a serious threat to the public or environment unless handled recklessly;
4. the risk from disposal of pharmaceuticals is low provided it is properly handled;
5. pharmaceutical disposal should be undertaken at minimum financial cost and with minimum risk to public health and the environment considering the local circumstances;
6. disposal of pharmaceuticals should be carried out under the supervision of regional and national authorities, who organize it according to strict criteria; it must not be carried out by individuals.

Information on pharmaceutical disposal must be carefully handled as it may be politicized and sensationalized. If the public and media are not kept judiciously informed of the efforts to dispose of expired pharmaceuticals safely, the disposal work may be severely hampered by misinformation propagated by uninformed journalists and politicians. Good public relations, including comprehensive dissemination of information, is, therefore, an important element in achieving satisfactory safe disposal.

2. Disposal Methods

Constraints in funding for disposal of waste pharmaceuticals necessitate cost- effective management and methods. The main way to achieve this is to sort the material to minimize the need for expensive or complicated disposal methods. Pharmaceutical sorting categories are described in Section 3 and the recommended disposal methods for each pharmaceutical sorting category in Section 4. Firstly however, the various disposal methods are briefly described here and summarized in Table 1.

2.1 *Return to Donor or Manufacturer*

Wherever practical the possibility of returning unusable drugs for safe disposal by the manufacturer should be explored; particularly drugs which present disposal problems, such as antineoplastics. For unwanted, unrequested donations, especially those that arrive past or unreasonably near their expiry date, it may be possible to return them to the donor for disposal.

Cross–Frontier Transfer of Pharmaceutical Waste

There are currently no international conventions regulating transfer of pharmaceutical products across frontiers. However, expired or spoiled pharmaceuticals are considered as hazardous waste and as such, if transferred across frontiers, become regulated and subject to the Basel Convention on the Transfrontier Shipment of Hazardous Wastes. This involves prescribed procedures to obtain permission to cross international borders along the transit route prior to actual transport. These procedures can take several months to complete.

2.2 *Landfill*

To landfill means to place waste directly into a land disposal site without prior treatment or preparation. Landfill is the oldest and the most widely practiced method of disposing of solid waste. Three types are recognized.

Open Uncontrolled Non-Engineered Dump

A non-engineered dump is probably the most common land disposal method in developing countries. Untreated waste discharged into an uncontrolled, non- engineered open dump does not protect the local environment and should not be used. Discarding of untreated waste pharmaceuticals into such a site is not recommended except as a last resort. They should preferably be discharged after immobilization by encapsulation or inertization. As a last resort, where it is not possible to immobilize the waste pharmaceuticals, then the untreated wastes must be covered rapidly with large quantities of municipal waste to prevent scavenging. It should be noted that discarding in open, uncontrolled dumps with insufficient isolation from the aquifer or other watercourses can lead to pollution, with the risk of drinking water contamination in the worst cases.

Engineered Landfill

Such a landfill has some features to protect from loss of chemicals into the aquifer. Direct deposit of pharmaceuticals is second best to discharging immobilized pharmaceutical waste into such a landfill.

Highly Engineered Sanitary Landfill

Properly constructed and operated landfill sites offer a relatively safe disposal route for municipal solid wastes, including waste pharmaceuticals. The top priority is protection of the aquifer. An appropriate landfill consists of an evacuated pit isolated from watercourses and above the water table. Each day's solid waste is compacted and covered with soil to maintain sanitary conditions. The term "safe sanitary landfill" refers to such a site that is adequately situated, constructed and managed. Upgrading an uncontrolled waste disposal site to a reasonable standard should be considered, and advice is available from WHO.

2.3 *Waste Immobilization: Encapsulation*

Encapsulation involves immobilizing the pharmaceuticals in a solid block within a plastic or steel drum. Drums should be cleaned prior to use and should not have contained explosive or hazardous materials previously. They are filled to 75% capacity with solid and semi-solid pharmaceuticals, and the remaining space is filled by pouring in a medium such as cement or cement/lime mixture, plastic foam or bituminous sand. For ease and speed of filling, the drum lids should be cut open and bent back. Care should be taken to avoid cuts to hands when placing pharmaceuticals in the drums. Once the drums are filled to 75% capacity, the mixture of lime, cement and water in the proportions 15:15:5 (by weight) is added and the drum filled to capacity. A larger quantity of water may be required sometimes to attain a satisfactory liquid consistency. Steel drum lids should then be bent back and sealed, ideally by seam or spot welding. The sealed drums should be placed at the base of a landfill and covered with fresh municipal solid waste. For ease of movement, the drums may be placed on pallets which can then be put on a pallet transporter.

Encapsulation of antineoplastic drugs requires a slightly different technique (see Section 4.6).

2.4 *Waste Immobilization: Inertization*

Inertization is a variant of encapsulation and involves removing the packaging materials, paper, cardboard and plastic, from the pharmaceuticals. Pills need to be removed from their blister packs. The pharmaceuticals are then ground and a mix of water, cement and lime added to form a homogenous paste. Worker protection in the form of protective clothing and masks is required as there may be a dust hazard. The paste is then transported in the liquid state by concrete mixer truck to a landfill and decanted into the normal urban waste. The paste then sets as a solid mass dispersed within the municipal solid waste. The process is relatively inexpensive and can be carried out with unsophisticated equipment. The main requirements are a grinder or road roller to crush the pharmaceuticals, a concrete mixer, and supplies of cement, lime and water.

The approximate ratios by weight used are as follows:

- pharmaceutical waste : 65%
- lime : 15%
- cement : 15%
- water : 5% or more to form a proper liquid consistency.

2.5 *Sewer*

Some liquid pharmaceuticals, e.g. syrups and intravenous (IV) fluids, can be diluted with water and flushed into the sewers in small quantities over a period of time without serious public health or environmental affect. Fast flowing watercourses may likewise be used to flush small quantities of well-diluted liquid pharmaceuticals or antiseptics. The assistance of a hydrogeologist or sanitary engineer may be required in situations where sewers are in disrepair or have been war damaged.

2.6 *Burning in Open Containers*

Pharmaceuticals should not be destroyed by burning at low temperature in open containers, as toxic pollutants may be released into the air. Paper and cardboard packaging, if they are not to be recycled, may be burnt. Polyvinyl chloride (PVC) plastic however must not be burnt. While burning pharmaceutical waste is not advocated as a method of disposal, it is recognized that it is not infrequently used. It is strongly recommended that only very small quantities of waste pharmaceuticals be disposed of in this way.

2.7 *Medium Temperature Incineration*

In many countries there are no high temperature, two–chamber incinerators designed to handle more than 1% halogenated compounds. Such incinerators meet strict emission control standards, such as those published by the European Union. However, it is likely that only medium temperature furnaces and incinerators will be available. In emergency situations the responsible authorities may consider it acceptable to treat expired solid form pharmaceuticals using a two–chamber incinerator that operates at the minimum temperature of 850°C, with a combustion retention time of at least two seconds in the second chamber. Many older municipal solid waste incinerators are medium temperature incinerators and the use of these facilities is encouraged as an interim measure, rather than less safe options, such as inadequate discharge to a landfill. In this case, it is recommended that the pharmaceutical waste is diluted with large quantities of municipal waste (approximately 1:1000). Such incinerators are not designed to incinerate halogenated compounds safely. The very low halogen content in most pharmaceuticals is likely to result in negligible halogen content in the combustion gases.

Halogen Content of Pharmaceutical Waste

Pharmaciens Sans Frontières, working in Bosnia (Mostar), found the halogen content of donated pharmaceuticals for disposal to be very low; well below the maximum permissible values for incinerators/ plants licensed for non-halogen wastes in the European Union.

2.8 *High Temperature Incineration Using Existing Industrial Plants*

Industries which use high temperature technology, such as cement kilns, coal fired thermal power stations or foundries, usually have furnaces that operate at temperatures well in excess of 850°C, have long combustion retention times and disperse exhaust gases via tall chimneys, often to high altitudes. Many countries do not possess and cannot justify economically, expensive and sophisticated chemical waste disposal facilities, so the use of an industrial plant provides a viable and cheap alternative.

Cement kilns are particularly suited for the disposal of expired pharmaceuticals, chemical waste, used oil, tyres, etc. Several features of cement kilns make them suitable for pharmaceutical disposal. During burning the cement raw materials reach temperatures of 1450°C, while the combustion gases reach temperatures up to 2000°C. The gas residence time at these high temperatures is several seconds. In these conditions all organic waste components are effectively disintegrated. Some potentially dangerous or toxic combustion products become adsorbed into the cement clinker product or are removed in the heat exchange equipment.

Cement producers in many countries are keen to use alternative fuels, as their use reduces the fuel bill without adversely affecting the quality of the cement. With appropriate environmental impact control mechanisms in place there will be even less impact on the surrounding area. It is recommended that discussions be held with cement companies and the appropriate environmental agencies to arrange for waste to be disposed of using a cement kiln.

Pharmaceuticals should be introduced into the furnace as a reasonably small proportion of the total fuel feed. It is suggested that as a sensible "rule of thumb" no more than 5% of the fuel fed into the furnace at any one time is pharmaceutical material. Cement kilns typically produce 1,500 to 8,000 metric tons of cement per day and therefore quite large quantities of pharmaceutical material can be disposed of in a short period. It may be necessary to remove packaging and/or to grind the pharmaceuticals to avoid clogging and blockage of the fuel feed mechanisms.

Annex I gives more details of European Community regulations on high temperature incineration of hazardous wastes. Incinerators conforming to these regulations may be used for the disposal of halogenated compounds, X-ray contrast media and povidone iodine; lower temperature incinerators should not be used.

2.9 *Chemical Decomposition*

If an appropriate incinerator is not available, the option of chemical decomposition can be used in accordance with the manufacturer's recommendations, followed by landfill. This method is not recommended unless chemical expertise is readily available. Chemical inactivation is tedious and time consuming, and stocks of the chemicals used in treatment must be made available at all times. For disposal of a small quantity of antineoplastic drugs this method may be practical. However for large quantities, for example, more than 50 kg of antineoplastics, chemical decomposition is not practical, as even small consignments need to be treated through repeated application of this method.

Table 1: Summary of Disposal Methods in and After Emergencies

Disposal Methods	*Types of Pharmaceutical*	*Comments*
Return to donor or manufacturer, transfrontier transfer for disposal	All bulk waste pharmaceuticals, particularly antineoplastics.	Usually not practical - transfrontier procedures may be time consuming.
High temperature incineration with temperatures greatly in excess of 1200°C.	Solids, semisolids, powders, antineoplastics, controlled substances.	Expensive, particularly for purpose-built incinerators. Use of existing industrial plants may be more practical.
Medium temperature incineration with two–chamber incinerator with minimum temperature of 850°C. Cement kiln incineration	In the absence of high temperature incinerators, solids, semi-solids, powders. Controlled substances.	Antineoplastics best incinerated at high temperature.
Immobilization Waste encapsulation	Solids, semi-solids, powders, liquids, antineoplastics, controlled substances.	
Inertization	Solids, semi-solids, powders, antineoplastics, controlled substances.	
Landfill Highly engineered sanitary landfill	Limited quantities of untreated solids, semi-solids and powders. Disposal of waste pharmaceuticals after immobilization preferable. PVC plastics.	

Disposal Methods	*Types of Pharmaceutical*	*Comments*
Engineered landfill	Waste solids, semi-solids and powders, preferably after immobilization. PVC plastics.	
Open uncontrolled non-engineered dump	As last resort untreated solids, semi- solids, powders – **must** be covered immediately with municipal waste. **Immobilization** of solids, semi-solids, powders **is preferable.**	Not for untreated controlled substances.
Sewer	Diluted liquids, syrups, intravenous fluids, small quantities of diluted disinfectants (supervised).	Antineoplastics, and undiluted disinfectants and antiseptics not recommended.
Fast–flowing watercourse	Diluted liquids, syrups, intravenous fluids; small quantities of diluted disinfectants (supervised).	Antineoplastics, and undiluted disinfectants and antiseptics not recommended.
Burning in open containers	As last resort, packaging, paper, cardboard.	Not acceptable for PVC plastics or pharmaceuticals.
Chemical decomposition	Not recommended unless special chemical expertise and materials available.	Not practical for quantities over 50 kg.

3. Sorting Categories

3.1 *The Objectives of Sorting*

The objective of sorting is to separate the pharmaceuticals into categories that require different disposal methods. The appropriate safe disposal method recommended will depend principally on the pharmaceutical dosage form of the drugs. Segregated temporary storage areas or receptacles must be provided for each sorted category.

Practical Advice on Sorting

Sorting involves an initial overall evaluation of the stockpile and subsequent division of pharmaceuticals into those suitable for use and those to be discarded. For those to be discarded a decision is made on the best method of disposal. To be efficient items should only be handled once. Pharmaceuticals suitable for use should remain in their packaging. The pharmaceuticals to be discarded should, when necessary, be separated from their packaging as late in the process as possible.

The sorting process includes:

- identifying each item;
- making a decision on whether it is usable;
- if usable, leaving packaging intact;
- if not usable, making a judgement on the optimal method of disposal and sorting accordingly;
- leaving packages and boxes intact until reaching their location, prior to definitive disposal or transport to an institution for use.

3.2 *Optimum Conditions for Sorting*

Sorting should be done in the open or in a well ventilated and, if necessary, heated covered structure designated by the local authority. Sorting should be done as close as possible to the stockpile in an orderly way, with all sorted material clearly labelled and separated at all times. Staff supplied with protective equipment (gloves, boots, overalls, dust masks, etc.), should work under the direct supervision of a pharmacist. They should receive training on the sorting criteria, and health and safety risks associated with handling the materials.

Once sorted, the pharmaceuticals should be carefully packed into steel drums or into containers such as sturdy cardboard boxes, with the contents clearly indicated on the outside of the containers. The materials should be kept in a dry secure and preferably separate room to avoid being confused with in–date pharmaceuticals, until disposal is carried out.

3.3 *Sorting Categories*

The top priority of the sorting process is to separate out the pharmaceuticals that are categorized as controlled substances (e.g. narcotics), antineoplastic (cytotoxic- anti–cancer) drugs and any other hazardous non-pharmaceutical products that may have been mixed among the pharmaceuticals. These must all be stored in separate, secure designated areas prior to their separate, safe disposal.

The remaining unwanted pharmaceuticals must be further sorted into different categories by dosage form, (capsules, powders, solutions, suppositories, syrups, tablets). The following sorting categories and subcategories are suggested.

3.4 *Pharmaceuticals and Other Materials which can Still be Used*

A large proportion of the volume of a typical stockpile of waste drugs is not occupied by the pharmaceuticals themselves, but rather by other items, such as medical material and equipment, food, clothing, boxes, pallets, and general rubbish. The first step in dealing with these stockpiles is to remove and dispose of these non-drug, non-chemical items. All such items should be clearly separated from pharmaceuticals and chemicals.

Non-pharmaceutical useful materials

Medical equipment, beds, wheelchairs, dressings, clothing, laboratory glassware, etc. can either be utilized by the institution or by other facilities, recycled, cannibalized for spare parts or disposed to a landfill.

Useful pharmaceuticals

If feasible, pharmaceuticals within their expiry date and considered useful should be separated out and immediately used by the institution or reallocated according to the needs and instructions of the regional health authorities. A list can be prepared giving details of the items available, quantities and expiry dates and circulated to others who can use the materials. While this separation is logical and appealing, experience indicates that it may not always be an efficient use of time and resources.

Chemicals

Acids, alkalis, reagents, phenol-based chemicals used for cleaning floors, disinfectants, etc. can be put to good use. If large quantities of these items are found a list may be prepared and offered to other potential users, such as hospitals, universities, or school laboratories, etc.

3.5 *Expired or Unwanted Pharmaceuticals*

Pharmaceuticals that should never be used and should always be considered as *pharmaceutical waste are:*

- all expired pharmaceuticals;
- all unsealed syrups or eye drops (expired or unexpired);
- all cold chain damaged unexpired pharmaceuticals that should have been stored in a cold chain but were not (for example: insulin, polypeptide hormones, gamma globulins and vaccines);
- all bulk or loose tablets and capsules. If unexpired these should only be used when the container is still sealed, properly labelled or still within the original unbroken blister packs;
- all unsealed tubes of creams, ointments, etc. (expired or unexpired).

Special disposal is needed for the following:

- controlled substances; e.g. narcotics, psychotropic substances;
- anti-infective drugs;
- antineoplastics;
- cytotoxic-anti–cancer drugs, toxic drugs;
- antiseptics and disinfectants.

For more information refer to Sections 4.4, 4.5, 4.6 and 4.7.

All other pharmaceuticals should be sorted by dosage form:

solids, semi-solids and powders

- tablets, capsules, granules, powders for injection, mixtures, creams, lotions, gels, suppositories, etc.;

liquids

- solutions, suspensions, syrups, etc.;
- ampoules;

aerosol canisters

- including propellant-driven sprays and inhalers.

3.6 *Hazardous or Potentially Hazardous Non-pharmaceutical Materials*

All non-pharmaceutical, potentially dangerous waste such as chemicals, cleaning solutions, batteries and waste oil must be dealt with on a case-by-case basis by the hazardous waste expert. They must not be handled by the pharmaceutical teams unless expressly directed to do so. This waste requires separate and careful labelling and storage until disposal.

3.7 *Recyclable Material*

Waste paper, cloth, packing materials, clothes, gauze and wooden items, such as pallets, can be recycled, burned or disposed of as normal waste to a landfill. Plastic, metal and glass items can be reused (glassware can be given to laboratories, mechanical items given to scrap dealers), recycled (if facilities are available) or disposed of in a landfill. Depending on the type of material and its proposed reuse, appropriate treatment, such as cleaning or disinfection, may be needed. Other general rubbish can be disposed of in a landfill. If a recycling programme exists for the reuse of such materials they can be separated from the pharmaceuticals prior to their disposal in the landfill.

4. Recommended Disposal Methods

by Sorting Category

4.1 *Solids, Semi-Solids and Powders Anti-infective Drugs, Controlled Drugs and Antineoplastics*

If it is not possible to return these to the manufacturer or adequate incineration is unavailable then encapsulation or inertization is recommended before discharge to a landfill (refer to Sections 4.4, 4.5 and 4.6). Anti-infective drugs and antineoplastics are encapsulated to delay release to the environment and avoid high concentrations. Controlled drugs should be immobilized under supervision of the pharmacist, the police or a judicial representative, depending on the local regulations.

Other Drugs

Small quantities of solid and semi-solid pharmaceuticals, typically not more than 1% of the total daily waste, can be disposed of directly in a landfill with large volumes of municipal solid waste, if no other suitable method is available. The figure of 1% is based on expert opinion rather than scientific evidence. It is further postulated that in emergencies and situations where the stockpile is large (many hundreds of tons), then 5-10% of the total daily municipal waste would be an acceptable daily disposal figure, where disposal of municipal waste is greater than 50 metric tons per day. In this case the landfill should be well managed and the disposal should be for a fixed period of time.

The pharmaceutical solid waste should be disposed of at the base of the working face of the landfill and covered immediately by fresh municipal waste. Security measures to prevent scavenging should be in place. Pharmaceuticals classed as readily biodegradable organic material in the solid or semi-solid form, e.g. vitamins, can also be disposed of in a landfill.

Large quantities of solid and semi-solid pharmaceuticals are best destroyed by high temperature incineration as previously described. Medium temperature incineration is however widely practiced for solid form pharmaceuticals, provided that the pharmaceuticals are "diluted" in large quantities of municipal waste. Many countries however do not have access to either high or medium temperature incineration plants, and the use of the encapsulation method represents an acceptable, but not always feasible, method of disposal for large quantities of pharmaceuticals.

Procedure

Solids, semi-solids and powders should be removed from their outer packaging but remain in their inner packaging and placed in clean plastic or steel drums, for treatment according to the encapsulation method. Removing outer packaging dramatically reduces the volume for disposal for methods such as encapsulation. Small quantities of pharmaceuticals still within their packaging may be discharged into a landfill as described above. They should be immediately covered with municipal waste. Outer packaging should be disposed of as non-drug, non-chemical materials by recycling or burning.

The separation of materials should be as follows:

- tablets and capsules in plastic/foil blisters should be removed from all outer packaging but not from blisters;
- tablets and capsules in bottles should be removed from outer packaging but not bottles;
- tablets and effervescents in tubes should be removed from outer packaging but not from tubes;
- powders in sachets or bottles should be removed from outer packaging but not from sachets or bottles.

Any large quantities of a single type of drug should be checked by the supervising pharmacist to ensure that the drug is not an anti-infective drug, antineoplastic or controlled substance. If the drug is an antineoplastic, it should be treated according to the procedure for antineoplastics outlined in Section 4.6. Controlled substances should be treated as normal solids, but with supervision according to local regulations. See Sections 4.3 and 4.4 for treatment of anti-infective drugs. Very large quantities of loose tablets should be mixed with other medicines in several different steel drums to avoid very high concentrations of a single drug in any one drum.

4.2 *Liquids Pharmaceuticals with No or Low Toxicity*

Pharmaceuticals that can be classed as readily biodegradable organic material include liquid vitamins that may be diluted and flushed into a sewer. Harmless solutions of different concentrations of certain salts, amino acids, lipids or glucose may also be disposed of in sewers.

Other Liquid Pharmaceuticals (except controlled drugs, antineoplastics or anti-infective drugs)

Small quantities of other liquid pharmaceuticals, which are not controlled substances, anti-infective drugs, or antineoplastics, can be flushed into sewers. If there are no sewers or there is no functioning sewage treatment plant, liquid pharmaceuticals can be first diluted with large volumes of water and poured into large watercourses, providing they are immediately dispersed and diluted by the flowing river water.

Liquid pharmaceutical waste may be disposed of using the cement encapsulation procedure (see Section 2.3), high temperature incineration or in cement kilns (see Section 2.8).

It is not acceptable to discharge liquid pharmaceuticals, diluted or not, into slow moving or stagnant surface waters.

4.3 *Ampoules*

These can be crushed on a hard impermeable surface (e.g. concrete) or in a metal drum or bucket using a stout block of wood or a hammer. Workers doing this should wear protective equipment, such as eye protection, boots, clothing and gloves. The crushed glass should be swept up, placed in a container suitable for sharp objects, sealed and disposed of in a landfill. The liquids released from the ampoules should be diluted and disposed of as described above.

Ampoules should not be burnt or incinerated as they will explode, possibly causing injury to operators and damage to the furnace or incinerator. Melted glass will also clog up the grate of a furnace or incinerator if the operating temperature is above the melting point of glass.

Volatile liquids in small quantities can be allowed to evaporate in the open air.

NB: Ampoules of antineoplastics or anti-infective drugs must not be crushed and the liquid discharged to sewers. They should be treated using the encapsulation or inertization disposal methods described above.

4.4 *Anti-infective Drugs*

Anti-infective drugs should not be discarded in an untreated form. Generally they are unstable and are best incinerated, and if that is not possible encapsulated or inertized. Liquid anti-infective drugs may be diluted in water, left for two weeks and disposed to the sewer.

4.5 *Controlled Substances*

Controlled substances must be destroyed under supervision of a pharmacist or the police depending on national regulations. Such substances must not be allowed into the public domain as they may be abused. They should either be rendered unusable, by encapsulation or inertization, and then dispersed among the municipal solid waste in a landfill, or incinerated.

4.6 *Antineoplastics*

Antineoplastic drugs, previously called cytotoxics or anti-cancer drugs, have the ability to kill or stop growth of living cells. They are used in the chemotherapy of cancer which is usually performed in specialized treatment centres. It is extremely unlikely that they would form part of an aid donation in emergencies. However, if unwanted and discharged into the environment they can have very serious effects, such as interfering with reproductive processes in various life forms. Their disposal must therefore be handled with care.

Antineoplastics should be segregated from other pharmaceuticals and kept separately in clearly marked containers with rigid walls[9]. They should ideally be safely packaged and returned to the supplier for disposal.

If this option is not possible they must be destroyed in a two-chamber incinerator which operates at a high temperature of at least 1200°C in the secondary chamber, and is fitted with gas cleaning equipment. An after-burner (i.e. the secondary chamber) is important for the destruction of cytotoxic waste, as it is possible that antineoplastic solutions could become aerosolized following the initial combustion in the primary chamber. As a result, without a higher temperature secondary chamber, degraded antineoplastic material may be emitted from the chimney. The secondary combustion chamber consequently ensures that such antineoplastic substances are fully incinerated.

Antineoplastic drugs/waste should never be disposed of in a landfill other than after encapsulation or inertization. Work teams handling these drugs must avoid crushing cartons or removing the product from its packages. They may only be discharged in a sewerage system after chemical decomposition and must not be discharged untreated into surface water drains or natural watercourses.

Special Treatment for Antineoplastics

For antineoplastics drums should be filled to 50% capacity with drugs, after which a well-stirred mixture of lime, cement and water in the proportions of 15:15:5 (by weight), should be added and the drums filled to capacity. A larger quantity of water may be required sometimes to attain a satisfactory liquid consistency. The drums should then be sealed by seam or spot welding and left to set for 7 to 28 days. This will form a firm, immobile, solid block in which the wastes are relatively securely isolated. The drums are then placed at the working face of a landfill which has been lined with an impermeable layer of clay or membrane.

Antineoplastic Drug Disposal

Methods of disposal:	1. return to supplier; 2. high temperature incineration
Methods of disposal of antineoplastics not to be used:	3. waste encapsulation; 4. low and medium temperature incineration; 5. disposal to sewers and water courses; 6. directly to landfill.

4.7 *Disinfectants*

In general disinfectants do not have an expiry date. They can be stored and gradually used over time so there is no real need to dispose of them. Large quantities of disinfectants must not be flushed into the sewer, as they may kill the bacteria in a sewage works and so stop the biological treatment of the sewage. Similarly large quantities should not be put into watercourses since the disinfectants will damage aquatic life. Small quantities of diluted disinfectant may be disposed of by discharge to a sewer providing the operation is supervised by a pharmacist and the quantities are strictly controlled to set limits. The guideline control proposed is 50 litres total per day, with the disposal spread over the whole working day.

If possible, disinfectants should be used, for example for toilet cleaning in hospitals. Some disinfectants with strong bactericidal and antiviral activity, such as Lysol (50% cresylic acid), may have an expiry date. If this date has passed, the material can still be used for general disinfection purposes at an appropriate dilution decided by a pharmacist, or disposed of in a chemical waste disposal facility or a cement kiln. Many countries do not have chemical waste disposal facilities, so the materials may have to be shipped out of the country. However this is an expensive and complicated operation and should only be contemplated if there is no viable alternative.

The World Health Organization publishes chemical safety sheets for common disinfectants and pesticides. The sheets provide data on the chemical composition of the substance and indicate suitable methods of disposal. The sheets may be obtained from WHO.

4.8 *Aerosol Canisters*

Disposable aerosol canisters and inhalers should not be burnt or incinerated, as high temperatures may cause them to explode, possibly causing injury to operators and/or damage to the furnace or incinerator. Provided they do not contain poisonous substances they should be disposed of in a landfill, dispersed among municipal solid wastes.

Table 2: Summary of Pharmaceutical Categories and Disposal Methods in and after Emergencies

Category	*Disposal Methods*	*Comments*
Solids	Landfill	No more than 1% of the daily municipal waste should be disposed of daily in an untreated form (non-immobilized) to a landfill.
Semi-solids	Waste encapsulation	
Powders	Waste inertization	
	Medium and high temperature incineration (cement kiln incinerator)	
Liquids	Sewer High temperature incineration (cement kiln incinerator)	Antineoplastics not to sewer.
Ampoules	Crush ampoules and flush diluted fluid to Sewer	Antineoplastics not to sewer.
Anti-infective drugs	Waste encapsulation Waste inertization	Liquid antibiotics may be diluted with water, left to stand for several weeks and discharged to a sewer.
	Medium and high temperature incineration (cement kiln incinerator)	
Antineoplastics	Return to donor or manufacturer Waste encapsulation Waste inertization Medium and high temperature incineration (cement kiln incinerator) (chemical decomposition)	Not to landfill unless encapsulated. Not to sewer. No medium temperature incineration.
Controlled drugs	Waste encapsulation Waste inertization Medium and high temperature incineration (cement kiln incinerator)	Not to landfill unless encapsulated.

Category	*Disposal Methods*	*Comments*
Aerosol canisters	Landfill Waste encapsulation	Not to be burnt: may explode.
Disinfectants	Use To sewer or fast–flowing watercourse: small quantities of diluted disinfectants (max. 50 litres per day under supervision)	No undiluted disinfectants to sewers or water courses. Maximum 50 litres per day diluted to sewer or fast–flowing watercourse. No disinfectants at all to slow moving or stagnant watercourses.
PVC plastic, glass	Landfill	Not for burning in open containers.
Paper, cardboard	Recycle, burn, landfill	